The Ɡ
Workout Plan

A Total Body Fitness Program for
Weight Training, Cardio, Core &
Stretching
By Dale L. Roberts
©2015

The 90-Day Home Workout Plan: A Total Body Fitness
Program for Weight Training, Cardio, Core & Stretching
All rights reserved
March 29, 2015
Copyright ©2015 One Jacked Monkey, LLC
onejackedmonkey.com
All photos courtesy of Kelli Rae Roberts, January 2015
Cover design by Sami Johnston. Cover image by
Depositphotos.com
ISBN-13: 978-1508865704
ISBN-10: 1508865701

My profound appreciation goes to:

Three of my biggest influences were in my early fitness development; David Moore for being such a positive role model and teaching me the fundamentals of weight training, Fraysher Ferguson (RIP) for being my inspiration and mentor when I needed it most, and, my old workout buddy, Shawn Knupp. Shawn, your early influence, competitive nature and friendship guided me to where I am today. I am forever grateful to you for being such a great friend.

And, my wife, Kelli, for your continued support in my fitness pursuits. Colleen Schlea for all your time and hard work you pour into editing my work.

Lastly, Christina Lucy and all the ladies at Code Pink Boot Camp in Phoenix. You were the inspiration behind this book and you may remember these workouts in great detail. Now you have them forever immortalized in print. Thanks for all your hard work, ladies!

DISCLAIMER

This book proposes a program of exercise recommendations. However, all readers must consult a qualified medical professional before starting this or any other health & fitness program. As with any exercise program, if at any time you experience any discomfort, pain or duress of any sort, stop immediately and consult your physician. The *90-day Home Workout Plan* is intended for an audience that is free of any health condition, physical limitation or injury. The creators, producers, participants, advertisers and distributors of this program disclaim any liabilities or losses in connection with the exercises or advice herein. Any equipment or workout area that is used should be thoroughly inspected ahead of use as free of danger, flaw or compromise. The user assumes all responsibility when performing any movements contained in this book and waives the equipment manufacturer, makers and distributors of the equipment of all liabilities.

Table of Contents

Introduction

There are millions of fitness books on the market, so what makes the *90-Day Home Workout Plan* any different? This book is a bit more unique since it is great for most fitness levels and can be used repeatedly. From the slightly experienced to the athletes, everyone can benefit from using the full workout plan with the in-depth descriptions of the exercises.

The best part of the *90-day Home Workout Plan* is you don't have to count repetitions. Though having a tally on how many reps you complete in a set time is great for comparison later, you still are not required to count. The workout is tough on its own, so adding rep counting to your workout can make it more difficult than it has to be.

These workouts are not just merely movement for movement's sake, but more of a specific movement-based program that will drive results in terms of body fat loss and muscle gain. Let's be clear, the muscle gain is not according to bodybuilding standards, so don't use this program if you are planning on competing in fitness. But, if you want to look leaner, feel better and accomplish more in less time, then this is your solution.

This workout plan is unique in that it covers all elements of physical fitness in about an hour. I'll discuss in the next chapter five specific components that make up each workout and the purpose of each in your fitness development. The goal of having them in all your workouts is to maximize the most out of the least amount of time.

The 90-day Home Workout Plan is designed to be fun, engaging and effective. You shouldn't have to feel obligated to workout or have to muster up the strength to get through yet another workout just because you feel you're required. Workouts should be the bright spot in your day, and that is what I have designed this program to be for you.

The 5 Components of the Workout

The 90-day Workout Plan has some predictability to it, yet changes regularly to keep your routine interesting and fun. The predictable parts of the workouts are the 5 components that are essential to a total body training program. A warm-up, cardio training, weight training, core development and stretching are the 5 components for a comprehensive approach to your fitness. But, every week the exercise program changes to keep you on your toes, keep your body guessing and keep your results coming.

Let's take a closer look at the importance of each component of a workout.

Component 1: Warm-up

The first 10 minutes of every workout is about moving the body, getting the blood pumping and mentally preparing yourself for the exercises ahead. Never skip this component, because the warm-up is crucial to get the most out of your routine, recover quicker and decrease the likelihood of injury[1].

For the 2 minutes, exercise slowly, then gradually increase your pace with each minute to the full 10 minutes. Your exercise pace should be enough that you can carry a conversation and start to break a sweat. Upon completion of your warm-up, avoid the temptation to procrastinate. Get into the very next component!

Component 2: Cardio

The primary objective of component 2 is to strengthen and to build endurance in your cardio-respiratory system, also known as your heart and your lungs. The heart is a muscle and much like any other muscle in the body, should be trained appropriately. If you can get your heart strong, you will gain more stamina, endurance and energy. With a strong heart, you'll be amazed how you much easier everything is, from your workouts to the most mundane chore. Cardio-respiratory training, or cardio, is appropriate for most everyone.

Increase your workout pace and really get moving in this

portion of the exercise routine. Your pace should be intense, filled with heavy breathing and having little ability to talk. On a scale of 0-10, 0 being no exertion and 10 being completely breathless, you should be between 6-8 rating[2]. Avoid exercising at an intensity of 10, because this can be detrimental to your health and you should never push yourself until you cannot breathe properly.

The scale is completely subjective, so don't compare your efforts or exertion to anyone else. Stay honest and continually re-evaluate your work with every exercise and workout.

Cardio is incorporated throughout the workout with the weight training and is sometimes the primary focus of a workout. In the average hour, the workout incorporates cardio from 10-15 minutes. If your weight training is faster paced, you may be able to achieve cardio training. The only time the workout should not be cardio-based is during your warm-up and in the latter portion of your routine. I cover this further in the final two components.

Component 3: Weight Training

The third component is developing your muscle through weight training. These exercises are designed to get you more toned, firm and to become an efficient fat-burning machine.

Think of your muscles as the cogs in your fat-burning furnace. The more muscle you have, the more it aids at fat loss. While you cannot firm up excess or loose skin, a good amount of muscle can get rid of extra jiggle, flabby arms, muffin top or baby belly. It's just a matter of being consistent and challenging yourself in every workout. One issue you cannot resolve with your exercise is to firm excess skin.

When you start this 90-day plan, you should use light weights. Five pound dumbbells are excellent to begin with, then gradually increase to heavier weights if your body adapts good enough between one week and the next. You will see your strength improve over the first 30 days and increase with each month after that. Your weights should be heavy enough to where you are breathing heavily at the end of an exercise. If you tire out before the exercise set is through, then go to lighter weights.

You may find you can handle a heavier weight with one exercise, but unable to use the same weight in another exercise. Where one muscle or set of muscles may handle a weight, other supportive muscles may still be adapting to that volume. It's better to be cautious and lift lighter on all parts, than to lift heavy at the detriment of the weaker parts.

For instance, you may be able to easily curl five-pound dumbbells, but you notice that if you combine that exercise with a squat that you feel a tightness in your low back. This may indicate your core has not adapted to that weight or that you are performing the movement improperly.

The exercise glossary in the back of the book gives you proper technique and tips to make each exercise effective. Constantly evaluate how you feel and where you feel it. Compare your performance from one week to the next to see if you should increase or decrease your efforts on a given exercise.

The same rule applies to this weight training as it does to cardio. Your exercise exertion should measure 6-8 on a scale of 0-10. Every repetition should have a steady pace.

Focus on breathing consistently and never hold your breath. You need to constantly provide your working muscles with oxygen-rich blood for you to function at your best. Without oxygen, your muscles will not adequately work. Breathe out each time you exert yourself. Your breath should be finishing up when your exercise is halfway finished. Breathe in when you return to the exercise start position.

For example, in a push up, when you press away from the floor, breathe out. When you pause at the top position, you should have all your air exhaled. Then, as you descend to the ground, breathe in. The real test is properly breathing with every movement while performing proper technique. Breathing properly in an exercise can be tough to figure out, but remember:

-Exert = breathe out
-Pause = finish up the breath
-Release = breathe in

It's easy to forget about breathing while you are busy thinking about performing your exercise correctly. Perform your exercise slowly at first until you have mastered the movement and the breathing together.

Take a sip of water between each full set of exercises to keep you hydrated. This also recharges you mentally to attack the next round of exercises. Pace yourself in your weight training, because this is where you will spend a majority of your routine (15-20 minutes).

Every day, the programming changes to complement a certain group of muscles to maximize the most out of the workout time. The most efficient way to burn calories is to use more of your body in each exercise. Integrated movements, or exercises that require groups of muscles to work together, develop functionality in strength endurance. Functional exercising trains your body to perform everyday activities easier and safer.[3]

The workouts include movements that squat, push, pull and utilize core power and stability. Focusing on these movements provides more results out of less time. With squat, push and pull, you move the body in an integrated fashion, therefore, building functional muscle for everyday habits, patterns and routines.

By using a different set of movements for everyday of the week, your body has time to repair, or recover, in areas you may have already used in a previous routine. Workout recovery is crucial for your body to function properly from one workout to the next. When you exercise too hard and too often with no time for recovery, Overtraining Syndrome can occur and you will be wearing your body down rather than building it up[4]. To avoid any setbacks or injuries, you will be using a different group of muscles or exercising differently every workout.

For instance, your movements are squat for Monday, so come Tuesday and Wednesday, you may feel sore in your legs and abs. Tuesday and Wednesday would focus on a push or a pull movement routine, so that your legs have time to repair, heal and recover.

I recommend taking at least two days off per week from this routine to allow your body full recovery. On those days off, you should stay active and stretch any sore muscles in your free time to better prepare you for the next week's workouts[5].

With five days of training per week, this leaves very little to do other than repeat squat, push and pull. That is why the days in between those types of movements are combination (i.e. Squat/push, squat/pull) and total body routines.

Component 4: Core

In this component, you should begin to slow down your exercises and steady your breathing. In the previous components, your effort is 6-8 on a scale of 0-10. You should now bring your efforts between 3 to 5. The fourth component, core, also known as the trunk, addresses the major muscles that move, support and stabilize your spine[6]. This includes the entire abdominal area from front wrapping all the way around to the back, then the small muscles along the spinal column. These muscles help you bend forward, stand up straight, bend backwards and sideways, twist, draw your stomach in and stabilize the spine during movement.

Each core exercise should be done at a slow pace of a 3-count exertion, 3-count hold and a 3-count release. Breathe as natural as possible since most of these movements test your will to push forward. When you feel your breathing or your heart rate increase, slow down or pause. This is when you should start to settle your breathing, slow your heart rate and cool down.

Component 4 lasts 10 minutes or less, depending largely on available time. If you find you go over in your cardio and weight training, cut time in the core component. A lot of movements address the core in some capacity. Core exercises are featured throughout the workout, even beyond the typically expected bunch of crunches.

Component 5: Stretch

The last component, stretching, is the most vital step in cooling down, carrying on with your day and setting up for better recovery for the next workout. Don't overlook stretching, because this is the key to injury prevention and faster workout recovery[7].

Exercises tend to tighten and to restrict muscle movement,

and stretching alleviates tension and improves range of motion. The wider the range of motion in a muscle and joint, the more benefits you gain from each movement. The more range of motion you have in each of your joints, the deeper and longer a movement can be performed. More joint mobility brings better exercising and more calories burned per movement[8].

Not to mention, proper stretching is the best way to decrease your chances of injury[9]. If a muscle is excessively tight and trained repeatedly without any relief, that muscle is more susceptible to injury. Sometimes the smallest muscles can be strained, too, due to the surrounding larger muscles being over-stressed. If a large muscle is sore, over-trained or tired, then other muscles make up the difference. This adaptation cannot be consciously controlled; the body automatically does what it has to for survival or continued function, regardless of the potential outcome or detriment.

Hold each stretch twice for 15 seconds each while focusing on the specific muscle stretched. Be purposeful and slow in your breathing. Unwind, let your mind relax and reflect on your routine. Avoid letting your mind wander to your day ahead and stay in the moment of deepening each stretch so that it is uncomfortable yet not painful.

If you challenge yourself by getting deeper into a stretch, you will see vast improvements in your strength and endurance gains. Every inch you can stretch deeper is a victory, just like any weight lost, size change, or muscle gain. Stretching is integral in your overall physical development. Keep it up and use stretching many times outside of your workout.

Tips & Suggestions

Plan a few things ahead of your workouts. Here are some items to consider:

1) Turn off your TV
2) Turn off your phone, unless you are using it for the workout
3) Remove any distractions for the next hour

4)   Review your workout. If you can't remember it, keep it easily accessible

5)   Keep a clock or stopwatch for timing your exercises. There are quite a few mobile apps that have programmable timers, test one ahead of your workout to avoid any problems during your routine.

You'll need a few items for your workout, but not all the equipment will be used for every workout. Refer to your workout of the day to determine if it's needed:

1)   Cold water - to keep you refreshed and hydrated

2)   Clean towel - in case of excess sweating

3)   Exercise mat - any kind of yoga mat or gymnastics mat

4)   Two dumbbells - start with five pounds and increase the weight depending on how well you handle them with each exercise

5)   Rubberband (or exercise band) - this typically can be found at most sporting goods stores. Any tubing that is relatively light resistance. Graduate to heavier resistance bands when your body adapts to the routine. If you purchase a new rubberband, try to get a set that comes with accessories like a door attachment and handles.

6)   Exercise bench - make sure it is sturdy and in good shape

If you are lacking the equipment for an exercise, here are a few modifications you can use:

1)   Dumbbells - use a water jug or bottle or a back pack

2)   Rubberbands - use dumbbells

3)   Bench - steps or a chair braced against a wall

4)   Jump rope - skip without the rope

5)   Exercise mat - beach towel

Consider a couple things before your begin this routine to really get great results. First, proper hydration and nutrition is key for you to get anywhere in your fitness goals. You really can't exercise your way out of a bad diet, so be sure you are fueling your body with proper nutrition. Also, carrying the right mindset and attitude is critical to you sticking to your goals as they pertain to this workout plan. If you aren't mentally prepared or have the right mindset before jumping into this, then chances are likely that when the going gets tough, you may walk away from this plan. I discuss the basics of hydration, nutrition, mindset and more in my publication *The 3 Keys to Greater Health & Happiness: The Beginner's Guide to Exercise, Diet & Mindset* (available at Amazon).

WARNING

If you are ever short of breath or are having difficulty breathing, slow down your pace, but never stop moving. Avoid stopping completely when you feel overwhelmed. Ease up a little and focus more on your breathing so that your heart and lungs can continue to pump oxygen-rich blood throughout your body. When you overexert yourself in your workout, you stress your heart and lungs beyond their capacity[10]. This causes shortness of breath when your heart and lungs cannot keep up with your workout pace. Over the next five to ten minutes when you start to breathe better, slowly increase your exertion, but keep it below your prior efforts.

If you ever feel light-headed, dizzy or nauseous, you should call your emergency response number or have someone seek medical attention for you immediately. These symptoms can be caused by dehydration, lack of nutrition, asthma, or worse yet, heart attack[11]. According to the American Heart Association, you should wait no more than three minutes to call for help[12], because emergency personnel have the knowledge and equipment to get your heart beating again if it has stopped[13]. Never wait and see how the symptoms change. Always err on the side of caution and get help right away.

Phase 1: Days 1-30

Every Monday - Total Body

WARM UP - 1 minute per exercise set - mid-paced - 10 minutes total	
1) Side Bend - left	6) Trunk Rotation
2) Side Bend - right	7) Knee Up - left
3) Front & Back Bend	8) Knee Up - right
4) Helicopter	9) Stationary Jog
5) Hands Together Side Bend	10) Jumping Jacks
CARDIO - fast-paced- 5 minutes total	
1) Run/Jog	
WEIGHT TRAINING - 1 minute per exercise - mid to fast-paced - 15 minutes total	
1) DB Squat	
2) DB Bent Row	
3) Push Up	
4) Crunches	
5) DB Walking Lunge	
6) DB Bent Reverse Fly	
7) DB Overhead Extension	
Rest 1 Minute (first time only), REPEAT circuit	
CARDIO - fast-paced- 3 minutes total	
1) Run/Jog	
WEIGHT TRAINING -1 minute per exercise - mid to fast-paced - 7 minutes total	
1) DB Squat	
2) DB Overhead Press	
3) DB Curl	
4) DB Trunk Rotation	
5) DB Sumo Squat	
6) DB Overhead Press - Alternating	
7) DB Curl - Alternating	
CORE - 1 minute per exercise - slow to mid-paced - 10 minutes total	
1) Crunch	6) Cross Crunch
2) Lying Leg Extension	7) Reverse Crunch
3) Bicycle Cross Crunch with leg hold	8) Russian Twist
4) Scissors	9) Flutters
5) Side to Side Crunch	10) Planks
STRETCH - hold twice for 30 seconds each - slow-paced - 10 minutes total	
1) Child Pose	6) Shoulder (wall) - right
2) Cobra Pose	7) Single Shoulder/Elbow Grasp -left
3) Kneeling Hip Flexor - left	8) Single Shoulder/Elbow Grasp - right
4) Kneeling Hip Flexor - right	9) Overhead Interlaced Palms
5) Shoulder (wall) - left	10) Neck ROM

Every Tuesday - Intervals

WARM UP - 1 minute per exercise set - mid-paced - 10 minutes total	
1) Side Bend - left	6) Trunk Rotation
2) Side Bend - right	7) Knee Up - left
3) Front & Back Bend	8) Knee Up - right
4) Helicopter	9) Stationary Jog
5) Hands Together Side Bend	10) Jumping Jacks
CARDIO - fast-paced- 5 minutes total	
1) Run/Jog ~2.5 minutes	
2) Shuttle Run (2:1 = work:rest) ~2.5 minutes	
INTERVAL TRAINING - fast-paced - 20 seconds on, 10 seconds off - 10 minutes total	
1) Jump Squat	1) Soccer Tap
2) Stationary Jog	2) Monkey Jacks
3) Jumping Jacks	3) Calf Bounce
4) Skaters	4) Jumping Lunge
REPEAT	REPEAT
REST 1 minute after each completed circuit	
CARDIO - fast-paced- 5 minutes total	
1) Jump Rope - 40 seconds	
2) Rest - 20 seconds	
REPEAT x4	
INTERVAL TRAINING - fast-paced - 20 seconds on, 10 seconds off - 10 minutes total	
1) Pop Squats	1) Monkey Jump
2) DB Uppercut	2) Knee Up - left
3) Explosive Side Lunge	3) Knee Up - right
4) Forward Jacks	4) Wall Climber
REPEAT	REPEAT
REST 1 minute after each completed circuit	
CORE - 1 minute each exercise set - slow to mid-paced - 10 minutes total	
1) Push Up Planks	6) Pumpers
2) Quadriped	7) Side Planks - left
3) Wall Chair	8) Side Lying Leg Lift - left
4) Floor Angel	9) Side Planks - right
5) Dynamic Bridge	10) Side Lying Leg Lift - right
STRETCH - hold twice for 30 seconds each - slow-paced - 10 minutes total	
1) Lying Ankle Pick - left	6) Shoulder (wall) - right
2) Lying Ankle Pick - right	7) Single Shoulder/Elbow Grasp - left
3) Single Calf (pike) - left	8) Single Shoulder/Elbow Grasp - right
4) Single Calf (pike) - right	9) Lateral Leg - left
5) Shoulder (wall) - left	10) Lateral Leg - right

Every Wednesday - Total Body

WARM UP - 1 minute per exercise set - mid-paced - 10 minutes total	
1) Side Bend - left	6) Trunk Rotation
2) Side Bend - right	7) Knee Up - left
3) Front & Back Bend	8) Knee Up - right
4) Helicopter	9) Stationary Jog
5) Hands Together Side Bend	10) Jumping Jacks
CARDIO - fast-paced- 5 minutes total	
1) Run/Jog	
WEIGHT TRAINING - 1 minute per exercise set - mid to fast-paced - 15 minutes	
1) DB Squat ~30 seconds	
2) DB Curl ~30 seconds	
3) DB Overhead press ~30 seconds	
4) DB Squat & Curl ~30 seconds	
5) DB Squat, Curl & Press ~30 seconds	
6) DB Reverse Lunge ~30 seconds	
7) DB Side Raise ~30 seconds	
8) DB Trunk Rotation ~30 seconds	
9) DB Walking Lunge & Side Raise ~30 seconds	
10) DB Walking Lunge with Side Raise & Trunk Rotation ~30 seconds	
REPEAT x2	
CARDIO - fast-paced- 5 minutes total	
1) Jump Rope - 40 seconds	
2) Rest - 20 seconds	
REPEAT x4	
CARDIO - fast-paced - 5 minutes total	
1) Shuttle Run (2:1 = work:rest)	
CORE -1 minute per exercise - slow to mid-paced - 10 minutes total	
1) Crunch	6) Dynamic Bridge
2) Cross Crunch	7) Quadriped
3) Leg Extension	8) Cherry Picker
4) Reverse Crunch	9) Pumpers
5) Side to Side Crunch	10) Planks
STRETCH - hold twice for 30 seconds each - slow-paced - 10 minutes total	
1) Child Pose	6) Single Shoulder/Elbow Grasp - left
2) Overhead Triceps - left	7) Single Shoulder/Elbow Grasp - right
3) Overhead Triceps - right	8) Forearm - left
4) Shoulder (wall) - left	9) Forearm - right
5) Shoulder (wall) - right	10) Neck ROM

Every Thursday - Intervals

WARM UP - 1 minute per exercise set - mid-paced - 10 minutes total	
1) Side Bend - left	6) Trunk Rotation
2) Side Bend - right	7) Knee Up - left
3) Front & Back Bend	8) Knee Up - right
4) Helicopter	9) Stationary Jog
5) Hands Together Side Bend	10) Jumping Jacks

CARDIO - fast-paced- 5 minutes total	
1) Run/Jog	

INTERVAL TRAINING - fast-paced - 20 seconds on, 10 seconds off - 10 minutes total	
1) Jump Rope	1) Jump Rope
2) Jumping Jacks	2) Explosive Side Lunge
3) Jump Rope	3) Jump Rope
4) Stationary Jog	4) Pop Squat
REPEAT	REPEAT
REST 1 minute after each completed circuit	

CARDIO - fast-paced- 5 minutes total	
1) Shuttle Run (2:1 = work:rest)	

INTERVAL TRAINING - fast-paced - 20 seconds on, 10 seconds off - 10 minutes total	
1) Monkey Jump	1) Knee Up - left
2) Jump Rope	2) Jump Rope
3) Skaters	3) Knee Up - right
4) Jump Rope	4) Jump Rope
REPEAT	REPEAT
REST 1 minute after each completed circuit	

CORE - slow to mid-paced - 1 minute each exercise set - 10 minutes total	
1) Crunch	6) Cherry Picker
2) Leg Extension	7) Legs Up Crunch
3) Window Wiper	8) Reverse Crunch with Leg Extension
4) Cross Crunch	9) Flutters
5) Reverse Crunch	10) Cross Arm & Leg Crunch

STRETCH - slow-paced - hold twice for 30 seconds each - 10 minutes total	
1) Knee Hug	6) Child Pose with Arm Thread - right
2) Lying Leg Extension Hold - left	7) Kneeling Hip Flexor - left
3) Lying Leg Extension Hold - right	8) Kneeling Hip Flexor - right
4) Child Pose with Arm Thread - left	9) Self Hug
5) Cobra Pose	10) Neck ROM

First Friday - Squat

WARM UP - 1 minute per exercise set - mid-paced - 10 minutes total	
1) Side Bend - left	6) Trunk Rotation
2) Side Bend - right	7) Knee Up - left
3) Front & Back Bend	8) Knee Up - right
4) Helicopter	9) Stationary Jog
5) Hands Together Side Bend	10) Jumping Jacks
CARDIO - fast-paced- 5 minutes total	
1) Shuttle Run (2:1 = work:rest)	
WEIGHT TRAINING -1 minute per exercise - mid to fast-paced - 10 minutes total	
1) DB Squat	
2) Single Leg Calf Raise - 1st set left, 2nd set right	
3) Jump Rope	
4) DB Lunge - 1st set left, 2nd set right	
5) Calf Bounce	
REPEAT	
CARDIO - fast-paced- 5 minutes total	
1) Run/Jog - 2 Minutes	
2) Jump Rope - 30 seconds, rest 30 seconds	
3) Sit Down - 30 seconds, rest 30 seconds	
4) Calf Bounce - 30 seconds, rest 30 seconds	
WEIGHT TRAINING - 1 minute per exercise - mid to fast-paced - 10 minutes total	
1) DB Sumo Squat	
2) DB Walking Lunge	
3) Jump Rope	
4) DB Step Up - 1st set left, 2nd set right	
5) Wall Chair	
REPEAT	
CORE - slow to mid-paced - 1 minute each exercise set - 10 minutes total	
1) Cross Crunch	6) Single Leg Dynamic Bridge - right
2) Dynamic Bridge	7) Floor Angel
3) Side to Side Crunch	8) Russian Twist
4) Single Leg Dynamic Bridge - left	9) Scissors
5) Reverse Crunch	10) Planks
STRETCH - hold twice for 30 seconds each - slow-paced - 10 minutes total	
1) Child Pose	6) Figure-4 - right
2) Knee Hug	7) Cross Leg Twist - left
3) Lying Leg Extension Hold - left	8) Cross Leg Twist - right
4) Lying Leg Extension Hold - left	9) Kneeling Hip Flexor - left
5) Figure-4 - left	10) Kneeling Hip Flexor - right

Second Friday - Push

WARM UP - 1 minute per exercise set - mid-paced - 10 minutes total	
1) Side Bend - left	6) Trunk Rotation
2) Side Bend - right	7) Knee Up - left
3) Front & Back Bend	8) Knee Up - right
4) Helicopter	9) Stationary Jog
5) Hands Together Side Bend	10) Jumping Jacks

CARDIO - fast-paced- 5 minutes total
1) Shuttle Run (2:1 = work:rest)

WEIGHT TRAINING -1 minute per exercise - mid to fast-paced - 10 minutes total
1) Push Up
2) DB Front Raise
3) DB Side Raise
4) DB Overhead Extension
5) DB Stick Up
6) Dip
7) DB Bent Kickback
8) DB Uppercut
9) DB Upright Row
10) Jumping Jacks

CARDIO - fast-paced- 5 minutes total
1) Run/Jog - 60 seconds
2) Jump Rope - 60 seconds
3) Soccer Tap - 30 seconds
REPEAT

WEIGHT TRAINING -1 minute per exercise - mid to fast-paced - 10 minutes total
1) Push Up - staggered - left over right
2) DB Lying Press
3) DB Lying Fly
4) DB Lying Pullover
5) REST
6) Push Up - staggered - right over left
7) DB Lying Press - alternating
8) DB Lying Fly - alternating
9) DB Lying Pullover - alternating
10) REST

CORE - slow to mid-paced - 1 minute each exercise set - 10 minutes total	
1) Crunch	6) Reverse Crunch
2) Leg Extension	7) Russian Twist
3) Window Wiper	8) Quadriped
4) Dynamic Floor Bridge	9) Jackknife
5) Cross Crunch	10) Planks

STRETCH - slow-paced - hold twice for 30 seconds each - 10 minutes total	
1) Child Pose	6) Shoulder (wall) - right
2) Cobra Pose	7) Single Shoulder/Elbow Grasp - left
3) Overhead Triceps - left	8) Single Shoulder/Elbow Grasp - right
4) Overhead Triceps - right	9) Reverse Hug
5) Shoulder (wall) - left	10) Neck ROM

Third Friday - Pull

WARM UP - 1 minute per exercise set - mid-paced - 10 minutes total	
1) Side Bend - left	6) Trunk Rotation
2) Side Bend - right	7) Knee Up - left
3) Front & Back Bend	8) Knee Up - right
4) Helicopter	9) Stationary Jog
5) Hands Together Side Bend	10) Jumping Jacks
CARDIO - fast-paced- 5 minutes total	
1) Run/Jog	
WEIGHT TRAINING - 1 minute per exercise - mid to fast-paced - 10 minutes total	
1) DB Bent Row	
2) DB Zottman Curl	
3) DB Bent Reverse Fly	
4) DB Side Raise	
5) Soccer Tap	
6) DB Bent Row - alternating	
7) DB Zottman Curl - alternating	
8) DB Bent Reverse Fly - alternating	
9) DB Side Raise - alternating	
10) Calf Bounce	
CARDIO - fast-paced- 5 minutes total	
1) Shuttle Run (2:1 = work:rest)	
WEIGHT TRAINING - mid to fast-paced - 5 minutes total	
1) RB Pulldown	
2) DB Bent Straight Arm Kickback	
3) RB Front Pulldown	
4) DB Bent Single Arm Row - 30 seconds left, 30 seconds right	
5) Soccer Tap	
CARDIO - fast-paced- 2.5 minutes total	
1) Shuttle Run	
CARDIO - fast-paced- 2.5 minutes total	
1) Run/Jog	
CORE - slow to mid-paced - 1 minute each exercise set - 10 minutes total	
1) Crunch	6) Jackknife
2) Reverse Crunch	7) Bicycle Cross Crunch
3) Bicycles	8) Russian Twist
4) Window Wiper	9) Cross Arm & Leg Crunch
5) Legs Up Crunch	10) Planks
STRETCH - slow-paced - hold twice for 30 seconds each - 10 minutes total	
1) Child Pose	6) Single Shoulder/Elbow Grasp - left
2) Cobra Pose	7) Single shoulder/Elbow Grasp - right
3) Reverse Hug	8) Forearm - left
4) Shoulder with Straight Arm (wall) - left	9) Forearm - right
5) Shoulder with Straight Arm (wall) - right	10) Overhead Arm Hold (wall)

Fourth Friday - Squat

WARM UP - 1 minute per exercise set - mid-paced - 10 minutes total	
1) Side Bend - left	6) Trunk Rotation
2) Side Bend - right	7) Knee Up - left
3) Front & Back Bend	8) Knee Up - right
4) Helicopter	9) Stationary Jog
5) Hands Together Side Bend	10) Jumping Jacks
CARDIO - fast-paced- 5 minutes total	
1) Jump Rope - 30 seconds	
2) Static Squat - 30 seconds	
REPEAT x4	
WEIGHT TRAINING - 1 minute per exercise - mid to fast-paced - 10 minutes total	
1) DB Single Leg Squat - left	
2) DB Single Leg Squat - right	
3) Single Leg Calf Raise - left	
4) DB Walking Lunge	
5) Single Leg Calf Raise - right	
REPEAT	
CARDIO - fast-paced- 2.5 minutes total	
1) Run/Jog	
WEIGHT TRAINING - mid to fast-paced - 1 minute per exercise - 10 minutes total	
1) DB Sumo Squat	
2) Reverse Lunge with Knee Up - left	
3) Reverse Lunge with Knee Up - right	
4) Calf Raise	
5) Calf Bounce	
CARDIO - fast-paced- 2.5 minutes total	
1) Shuttle Run (2:1 = work:rest)	
CORE - slow to mid-paced - 1 minute each exercise set - 10 minutes total	
1) Wall Chair	6) Reverse Crunch with Leg Extension
2) Lying Leg Extension	7) Planks with Alternating Leg Lift
3) Single Leg Dynamic Bridge - left	8) Side Planks - left
4) Reverse Crunch	9) Quadriped
5) Single Leg Dynamic Bridge - right	10) Side Planks - right
STRETCH - hold twice for 30 seconds each - slow-paced - 10 minutes total	
1) Child Pose	6) Figure-4 - right
2) Knees Hug	7) Cross Leg Twist - left
3) Single Leg Extension Hold - left	8) Cross Leg Twist - right
4) Single Leg Extension Hold - left	9) Kneeling Hip Flexor - left
5) Figure-4 - left	10) Kneeling Hip Flexor - right

Phase II: Days 31-60

First & Third Monday - Total Body

WARM UP - 1 minute per exercise set - mid-paced - 10 minutes total	
1) Side Bend - left	6) Trunk Rotation
2) Side Bend - right	7) Knee Up - left
3) Front & Back Bend	8) Knee Up - right
4) Helicopter	9) Stationary Jog
5) Hands Together Side Bend	10) Jumping Jacks
CARDIO - fast-paced- 2 minutes total	
1) Run/Jog	
WEIGHT TRAINING -1 minute per exercise - mid to fast-paced - 18 minutes total	
1) Jump Rope	
2) DB Walking Lunge	
3) RB Pulldown	
4) RB Triceps Extension	
REPEAT	
5) Jump Rope	
6) Single Leg Squat - left	
7) Single Leg Squat - right	
8) Push Up - bench	
9) Dip	
REPEAT	
CARDIO - fast-paced- 2 minutes total	
1) Shuttle Run (2:1 = work:rest)	
WEIGHT TRAINING - mid to fast-paced - 1 minute per exercise - 8 minutes	
1) Jump Rope	
2) DB Squat with Single Arm Cross Press - left	
3) DB Squat with Single Arm Cross Press - right	
4) DB Sumo Squat with Curl & Press	
REPEAT	
CORE - slow to mid-paced - 1 minute each exercise set - 10 minutes total	
1) Crunch	6) Cross Crunch
2) Lying Leg Extension	7) Reverse Crunch
3) Bicycle Cross Crunch with Leg Hold	8) Russian Twist
4) Scissors	9) Flutters
5) Side to Side Crunch	10) Planks
STRETCH - slow-paced - hold twice for 30 seconds each - 10 minutes total	
1) Child Pose	6) Seated Knee Hug - left
2) Kneeling Hip Flexor - left	7) Seated Knee Hug -right
3) Kneeling Hip Flexor - right	8) Self Hug
4) Seated Hamstring - left	9) Reverse Hug
5) Seated Hamstring - right	10) Neck ROM

First & Third Tuesday - Intervals

WARM UP - 1 minute per exercise set - mid-paced - 10 minutes total	
1) Side Bend - left	6) Trunk Rotation
2) Side Bend - right	7) Knee Up - left
3) Front & Back Bend	8) Knee Up - right
4) Helicopter	9) Stationary Jog
5) Hands Together Side Bend	10) Jumping Jacks
CARDIO - fast-paced- 3 minutes total	
1) Jump Rope - 30 seconds	
2) Static Squat - 30 seconds	
REPEAT x2	
INTERVAL TRAINING - fast-paced - 20 seconds on, 10 seconds off - 10 minutes total	
1) Jump Squat	1) Pop Squat
2) Jumping Lunge	2) Wall Climber
3) Soccer Tap	3) DB Uppercut
4) Skaters	4) Monkey Jump
5) Stationary Jog	5) Explosive Side Lunge
6) Calf Bounce	6) Forward Jacks
7) Jumping Jacks	7) Knee Up - left
8) Monkey Jacks	8) Knee Up - right
REST 1 minute after each completed circuit	
WEIGHT TRAINING - mid to fast-paced - 1 minute per exercise - 12 minutes	
1) RB Row	
2) Jump Rope	
3) RB High Row	
4) Soccer Tap	
5) RB Curl	
6) Explosive Side Lunge	
REPEAT	
CARDIO - fast-paced- 5 minutes total	
1) Run/Jog	
CORE - slow to mid-paced - 1 minute each exercise set - 10 minutes total	
1) Cross Crunch	6) Side to Side Crunch
2) Leg Lift	7) Cross Arm & Leg Crunch
3) Window Wiper	8) Bicycles
4) Legs Up Crunch	9) Cherry Picker
5) Leg Extension	10) Planks
STRETCH - slow-paced - hold twice for 30 seconds each - 10 minutes total	
1) Cat & Dog	6) Shoulder (wall) - left
2) Kneeling Hip Flexor - left	7) Shoulder (wall) -right
3) Kneeling Hip Flexor - right	8) Overhead Triceps - left
4) Single Calf (pike) - left	9) Overhead Triceps - right
5) Single Calf (pike) - right	10) Neck ROM

First & Third Wednesday - Squat

WARM UP - 1 minute per exercise set - mid-paced - 10 minutes total	
1) Side Bend - left	6) Trunk Rotation
2) Side Bend - right	7) Knee Up - left
3) Front & Back Bend	8) Knee Up - right
4) Helicopter	9) Stationary Jog
5) Hands Together Side Bend	10) Jumping Jacks

CARDIO - 30 seconds each exercise - fast-paced- 8 minutes total
1) Jump Rope
2) Static Squat
3) Jumping Jacks
4) Pump Lunge (switch legs each set)
REPEAT x3

WEIGHT TRAINING -1 minute per exercise - mid to fast-paced - 10 minutes total
1) DB Single Leg Squat - left
2) DB Single Leg Squat - right
3) DB Single Leg Calf Raise - left
4) DB Side Lunge
5) DB Single Leg Calf Raise - right
REPEAT

CARDIO - 30 seconds each exercise - fast-paced- 4 minutes total
1) Jump Rope
2) Static Squat
3) Jumping Jacks
4) Pump Lunge - 1st set: left, 2nd set: right
REPEAT

WEIGHT TRAINING - mid to fast-paced - 1 minute per exercise - 8 minutes total
1) DB Sumo Squat
2) DB Reverse Lunge with Knee Up - left
3) DB Reverse Lunge with Knee Up - right
4) Wall Chair with Toe Tap
REPEAT

CORE - slow to mid-paced - 1 minute each exercise set - 10 minutes total	
1) Crunch	6) Hip Thrust
2) Lying Leg Extension	7) Side Lying Leg Lift - left
3) Dynamic Bridge with Heel Raise	8) Side Lying Leg Lift - right
4) Jackknife	9) Quadriped
5) Legs Up Cross Crunch	10) Planks

STRETCH - slow-paced - hold twice for 30 seconds each - 10 minutes total	
1) Child Pose	6) Single Shoulder/Elbow Grasp - left
2) Overhead Triceps - left	7) Single Shoulder/Elbow Grasp - right
3) Overhead Triceps - right	8) Forearm - left
4) Shoulder (wall) - left	9) Forearm - right
5) Shoulder (wall) - right	10) Neck ROM

First & Third Thursday - Intervals

WARM UP - 1 minute per exercise set - mid-paced - 10 minutes total	
1) Side Bend - left	6) Trunk Rotation
2) Side Bend - right	7) Knee Up - left
3) Front & Back Bend	8) Knee Up - right
4) Helicopter	9) Stationary Jog
5) Hands Together Side Bend	10) Jumping Jacks
CARDIO - fast-paced- 10 minutes total	
1) Run/Jog - 5 minutes	
2) Shuttle Run (2:1 = work:rest) - 5 minutes	
INTERVAL TRAINING - fast-paced - 20 seconds on, 10 seconds off - 10 minutes total	
1) Jumping Jacks	1) Jump Rope
2) Pop Squat	2) Skaters
3) Push Up	3) Monkey Jacks
4) Wall Climber	4) Explosive Side Lunge
REPEAT	REPEAT
REST 1 minute after each completed circuit	
CARDIO - fast-paced- 10 minutes total	
1) Run/Jog - 2.5 minutes	
2) Shuttle Run (2:1 = work:rest) - 5 minutes	
3) Jump Rope - 2.5 minutes	
CORE - slow to mid-paced - 1 minute each exercise set - 10 minutes total	
1) Cross Crunch	6) Side to Side Crunch
2) Leg Lift	7) Cross Arm & Leg Crunch
3) Window Wiper	8) Bicycles
4) Legs Up Crunch	9) Cherry Picker
5) Leg Extension	10) Planks
STRETCH - slow-paced - hold twice for 30 seconds each - 10 minutes total	
1) Child Pose	6) Single Shoulder/Elbow Grasp - left
2) Overhead Triceps - left	7) Single Shoulder/Elbow Grasp - right
3) Overhead Triceps - right	8) Forearm - left
4) Shoulder (wall) - left	9) Forearm - right
5) Shoulder (wall) - right	10) Neck ROM

First & Third Friday - Push

WARM UP - 1 minute per exercise set - mid-paced - 10 minutes total	
1) Side Bend - left	6) Trunk Rotation
2) Side Bend - right	7) Knee Up - left
3) Front & Back Bend	8) Knee Up - right
4) Helicopter	9) Stationary Jog
5) Hands Together Side Bend	10) Jumping Jacks
CARDIO - fast-paced- 5 minutes total	
1) Run/Jog	
WEIGHT TRAINING -1 minute per exercise - mid to fast-paced - 13 minutes total	
1) Push Up	
2) DB Uppercut	
3) Dip	
4) DB Stick Up	
5) DB Overhead Extension	
6) Jumping Jacks	
Rest 1 Minute (first time only), REPEAT circuit	
CARDIO - fast-paced- 2 minutes total	
1) Run/Jog	
WEIGHT TRAINING - 1 minute per exercise set - mid-paced - 8 minutes total	
1) Push Up with Rotation	
2) DB Overhead Pull with Extension	
3) DB Arnold Press - alternating	
4) DB Bent Kickback - alternating	
5) DB Jab	
6) DB Cross	
7) DB Uppercut	
8) DB Back Fist	
CARDIO - fast-paced- 2 minutes total	
1) Run/Jog	
CORE - slow to mid-paced - 1 minute each exercise set - 10 minutes total	
1) Cross Crunch	6) Side Planks - left
2) Floor Angel	7) Side Planks - right
3) Side to Side Crunch	8) Superman
4) Pumpers	9) Quadriped
5) Russian Twist	10) Planks
STRETCH - slow-paced - hold twice for 30 seconds each - 10 minutes total	
1) Child Pose	6) Reverse Hug - left
2) Overhead Triceps - left	7) Single Shoulder/Elbow Grasp - left
3) Overhead Triceps - right	8) Single Shoulder/Elbow Grasp - right
4) Shoulder (wall) - left	9) Palms Interlaced Overhead
5) Shoulder (wall) - right	10) Neck ROM

Second & Fourth Monday - Total Body

WARM UP - 1 minute per exercise set - mid-paced - 10 minutes total	
1) Side Bend - left	6) Trunk Rotation
2) Side Bend - right	7) Knee Up - left
3) Front & Back Bend	8) Knee Up - right
4) Helicopter	9) Stationary Jog
5) Hands Together Side Bend	10) Jumping Jacks

CARDIO - fast-paced - 5 minutes total
1) Run/Jog

WEIGHT TRAINING - 1 minute per exercise - mid to fast-paced - 10 minutes total
1) DB Sit Down
2) DB Bent Row
3) Push Up
4) DB Step Up - left
5) DB Upright Row
6) DB Step Up - right
7) Dip
8) Calf Bounce
9) DB Curl & Press
10) DB Single Leg Squat with Curl (alternate legs)

CARDIO - fast-paced- 2.5 minutes total
1) Shuttle Run (2:1 = work:rest)

WEIGHT TRAINING - 1 minute per exercise - mid to fast-paced - 10 minutes total
1) DB Lying Press with Bridge
2) DB Lying Fly
3) DB Pullover with Bridge
4) Push Up - staggered - left over right
5) Push Up - staggered - right over left

CARDIO - fast-paced - 2.5 minutes total
1) Jump rope - 20 seconds
2) Rest - 10 seconds

REPEAT x4

CORE - 1 minute each exercise set - slow to mid-paced - 10 minutes total	
1) Crunch	6) Push Up Planks
2) Side to Side Crunch	7) Flutters
3) Window Wiper - legs extended	8) Russian Twist
4) Side Crunch - left	9) Coffin Sit Up
5) Side Crunch - right	10) Planks

STRETCH - slow-paced - hold twice for 30 seconds each - 10 minutes total	
1) Child Pose	6) Single Shoulder/Elbow Grasp - left
2) Overhead Triceps - left	7) Single Shoulder/Elbow Grasp - right
3) Overhead Triceps - right	8) Forearm - left
4) Shoulder (wall) - left	9) Forearm - right
5) Shoulder (wall) - right	10) Neck ROM

Second & Fourth Tuesday - Intervals

WARM UP - 1 minute per exercise set - mid-paced - 10 minutes total	
1) Side Bend - left	6) Trunk Rotation
2) Side Bend - right	7) Knee Up - left
3) Front & Back Bend	8) Knee Up - right
4) Helicopter	9) Stationary Jog
5) Hands Together Side Bend	10) Jumping Jacks
CARDIO - fast-paced - 5 minutes total	
1) Run/Jog - 2.5 minutes	
2) Shuttle Run (2:1 = work:rest) - 2.5 minutes	
INTERVAL TRAINING - fast-paced - 20 seconds on, 10 seconds off - 10 minutes total	
1) Jump Lunge	1) Skater
2) Calf Bounce	2) Jumping Jacks
3) Monkey Jacks	3) Stationary Jog
4) Soccer Tap	4) Jump Squat
REPEAT	REPEAT
REST 1 minute after each completed circuit	
CARDIO - fast-paced- 5 minutes total	
1) Jump Rope - 40 seconds	
2) Rest - 20 seconds	
REPEAT x4	
INTERVAL TRAINING - fast-paced - 20 seconds on, 10 seconds off - 10 minutes total	
1) Wall Climber	1) Forward Jacks
2) Knee Up - left	2) DB Uppercut
3) Knee Up - right	3) Explosive Side Lunge
4) Monkey Jump	4) Pop Squat
REPEAT	REPEAT
REST 1 minute after each completed circuit	
CORE - 1 minute each exercise set - slow to mid-paced - 10 minutes total	
1) Crunch	6) Pumpers
2) Bicycles	7) Side Planks - left
3) Russian Twist	8) Side Lying Leg Lift - left
4) Leg Lift	9) Side Planks - right
5) Side to Side Crunch	10) Side Lying Leg Lift - right
STRETCH - slow-paced - hold twice for 30 seconds each - 10 minutes total	
1) Standing Ankle Pick - left	6) Standing Hip Flexor - right
2) Standing Ankle Pick - right	7) Self Hug
3) Calf (wall) - left	8) Reverse Hug
4) Calf (wall) - right	9) Shoulder Roll
5) Standing Hip Flexor - left	10) Palms Interlaced Overhead

Second & Fourth Wednesday - Squat

WARM UP - 1 minute per exercise set - mid-paced - 10 minutes total	
1) Side Bend - left	6) Trunk Rotation
2) Side Bend - right	7) Knee Up - left
3) Front & Back Bend	8) Knee Up - right
4) Helicopter	9) Stationary Jog
5) Hands Together Side Bend	10) Jumping Jacks

CARDIO - 30 seconds per exercise - fast-paced - 5 minutes total	
1) Jump Rope	
2) Static Squat	
3) Jumping Jacks	
4) Pump Lunge - 1st set: left, 2nd set: right	
5) Explosive Side Lunges	
REPEAT	

WEIGHT TRAINING - 1 minute per exercise - mid to fast-paced - 10 minutes total	
1) Single Leg Squat - left	
2) Single Leg Squat - right	
3) Walking Lunge	
4) Single Leg Calf Raise - 1st set: left, 2nd set: right	
5) Sit Down	
REPEAT	

CARDIO - 30 seconds per exercise - fast-paced - 5 minutes total	
1) Jump Rope	
2) Static Squat	
3) Jumping Jacks	
4) Pump Lunge - 1st set: left, 2nd set: right	
5) Explosive Side Lunge	
REPEAT	

WEIGHT TRAINING - 1 minute per exercise - mid to fast-paced - 10 minutes total	
1) DB Sumo Squat	
2) DB Reverse Lunge with Knee Up - left	
3) Wall Chair with Toe Tap	
4) DB Reverse Lunge with Knee Up - right	
REPEAT	

CORE - 1 minute each exercise set - slow to mid-paced - 10 minutes total	
1) Crunch	6) Side to Side Crunch
2) Lying Leg Extension	7) Reverse Crunch
3) Bicycle Cross Crunch	8) Cherry Picker
4) Floor Angel	9) Scissors
5) Legs Up Cross Crunch	10) Planks

STRETCH - slow-paced - hold twice for 30 seconds each - 10 minutes total	
1) Child Pose	6) Single Shoulder/Elbow Grasp - left
2) Overhead Triceps - left	7) Single Shoulder/Elbow Grasp - right
3) Overhead Triceps - right	8) Forearm - left
4) Shoulder (wall) - left	9) Forearm - right
5) Shoulder (wall) - right	10) Neck ROM

Second & Fourth Thursday - Intervals

WARM UP - 1 minute per exercise set - mid-paced - 10 minutes total	
1) Side Bend - left	6) Trunk Rotation
2) Side Bend - right	7) Knee Up - left
3) Front & Back Bend	8) Knee Up - right
4) Helicopter	9) Stationary Jog
5) Hands Together Side Bend	10) Jumping Jacks
CARDIO - fast-paced - 5 minutes total	
1) Run/Jog - 2.5 minutes	
2) Shuttle Run (2:1 = work:rest) - 2.5 minutes	
INTERVAL TRAINING - fast-paced - 20 seconds on, 10 seconds off - 10 minutes total	
1) Monkey Jump	1) Calf Bounce
2) Stationary Jog	2) Monkey Jacks
3) Forward Jacks	3) Soccer Tap
4) Explosive Lateral Lunge	4) Jumping Lunge
REPEAT	REPEAT
REST 1 minute after each completed circuit	
CARDIO - fast-paced - 5 minutes total	
1) Jump Rope - 40 seconds	
2) Rest - 20 seconds	
REPEAT x4	
INTERVAL TRAINING - fast-paced - 20 seconds on, 10 seconds off - 10 minutes total	
1) DB Jab	1) Jumping Jacks
2) DB Cross	2) Knee Up - left
3) DB Uppercut	3) Knee Up - right
4) DB Back Fist	4) Stationary Jog
REPEAT	REPEAT
REST 1 minute after each completed circuit	
CORE - slow to mid-paced - 1 minute each exercise set - 10 minutes total	
1) Cross Crunch	6) Quadriped
2) Dynamic Bridge	7) Side Planks - left
3) Wall Chair	8) Side Lying Leg Lift - left
4) Floor Angel	9) Side Planks - right
5) Planks	10) Side Lying Leg Lift - right
STRETCH - slow-paced - hold twice for 30 seconds each - 10 minutes total	
1) Kneeling Hip Flexor - left	6) Shoulder (wall) - right
2) Kneeling Hip Flexor - right	7) Standing Hip Flexor - left
3) Single Calf (pike) - left	8) Standing Hip Flexor - right
4) Single Calf (pike) - right	9) Bent Hamstring - left
5) Shoulder (wall) - left	10) Bent Hamstring - right

Second & Fourth Friday - Pull

WARM UP - 1 minute per exercise set - mid-paced - 10 minutes total	
1) Side Bend - left	6) Trunk Rotation
2) Side Bend - right	7) Knee Up - left
3) Front & Back Bend	8) Knee Up - right
4) Helicopter	9) Stationary Jog
5) Hands Together Side Bend	10) Jumping Jacks

CARDIO - fast-paced - 5 minutes total
1) Run/Jog

WEIGHT TRAINING - 1 minute per exercise - mid to fast-paced - 10 minutes total
1) DB Bent Row - alternating
2) DB Stick Up - alternating
3) DB Curl - alternating
REPEAT
4) DB Upright Row & Curl
5) DB Front & Side Raise
6) DB Squatted Concentration Curl - 1st set: left, 2nd set: right
REPEAT

CARDIO - fast-paced- 5 minutes total
1) Run/Jog

WEIGHT TRAINING - 1 minute per exercise - mid to fast-paced - 10 minutes total
1) DB Bent Reverse Fly
2) DB Chicken Wing
3) DB Zottman Curl
4) DB Bent Overhand Row
5) DB Standing Preacher Curl - 1st set: left, 2nd set: right
REPEAT
6) RB Reverse Fly
7) RB Side Raise
8) RB 21s
9) RB Row
10) RB Hammer Curl
REPEAT

CORE - slow to mid-paced - 1 minute each exercise set - 10 minutes total	
1) Crunch	6) Cross Crunch
2) Reverse Crunch with Leg Extension	7) Reverse Crunch
3) Bicycle Cross Crunch with Leg Hold	8) Russian Twist
4) Scissors	9) Flutters
5) Side to Side Crunch	10) Planks

STRETCH - slow-paced - hold twice for 30 seconds each - 10 minutes total	
1) Child Pose	6) Single Shoulder/Elbow Grasp - left
2) Overhead Triceps - left	7) Single Shoulder/Elbow Grasp - right
3) Overhead Triceps - right	8) Forearm - left
4) Shoulder (wall) - left	9) Forearm - right
5) Shoulder (wall) - right	10) Neck ROM

Phase III: Days 61-90

First & Third Monday - Squat

WARM UP - 1 minute per exercise set - mid-paced - 10 minutes total	
1) Side Bend - left	6) Trunk Rotation
2) Side Bend - right	7) Knee Up - left
3) Front & Back Bend	8) Knee Up - right
4) Helicopter	9) Stationary Jog
5) Hands Together Side Bend	10) Jumping Jacks
CARDIO - 30 seconds per exercise - fast-paced - 5 minutes total	
1) Run/Jog - 30 seconds on, 30 seconds off	
REPEAT x4	
WEIGHT TRAINING - 1 minute per exercise - mid to fast-paced - 10 minutes total	
1) DB Single Leg Squat - alternating	
2) DB Transverse Lunge - alternating	
3) Static Squat with Heel Raise Hold	
4) Jumping Jacks	
5) DB Close Foot Squat	
REPEAT	
CARDIO - fast-paced - 5 minutes total	
1) Shuttle Run (2:1 = work:rest)	
WEIGHT TRAINING - 1 minute per exercise - mid to fast-paced - 10 minutes total	
1) DB Squat & Lunge	
2) DB Pumping Sumo Squat	
3) DB Side Lunge with Knee Up - 1st set: left, 2nd set: right	
4) Calf Bounce	
5) Monkey Jump	
REPEAT	
CORE - 1 minute each exercise set - slow to mid-paced - 10 minutes total	
1) Cross Leg Bridge - left	6) Side Lying Leg Lift - left
2) Coffin Sit Up	7) Quadriped
3) Cross Leg Bridge - right	8) Side Lying Leg Lift - right
4) Reverse Crunch with Leg Extension	9) Pumpers
5) Legs Up Crunch	10) Planks
STRETCH - hold twice for 30 seconds each - slow-paced - 10 minutes total	
1) Lying Knee Hug	6) Standing Bent Hamstring - right
2) Child Pose	7) Standing Cross Leg Glute - left
3) Kneeling Hip Flexor - left	8) Standing Cross Leg Glute - right
4) Kneeling Hip Flexor - right	9) Single Leg Calf (wall) - left
5) Standing Bent Hamstring - left	10) Single Leg Calf (wall) - right

First & Third Tuesday - Push

WARM UP - 1 minute per exercise set - mid-paced - 10 minutes total	
1) Side Bend - left	6) Trunk Rotation
2) Side Bend - right	7) Knee Up - left
3) Front & Back Bend	8) Knee Up - right
4) Helicopter	9) Stationary Jog
5) Hands Together Side Bend	10) Jumping Jacks

CARDIO - fast-paced- 5 minutes total	
1) Run/Jog	

WEIGHT TRAINING -1 minute per exercise - mid to fast-paced - 10 minutes total	
1) Push Up - staggered	
2) DB Jab	
3) Dip	
4) DB Cross	
5) DB Overhead Extension	
6) DB Uppercut	
7) Push Up - close grip - bench	
8) DB Back Fist	
9) DB Overhead Press - alternating	
10) DB Front & Side Raise	

CARDIO - fast-paced- 5 minutes total	
1) Run/Jog - 2.5 minutes	
2) Shuttle Run (2:1 = work:rest) - 2.5 minutes	

WEIGHT TRAINING - 1 minute per exercise set - mid-paced - 10 minutes total	
1) Push Up with Rotation	
2) DB Overhead Pull with Extension	
3) DB Arnold Press - alternating	
4) DB Bent Kickback - alternating	
5) Jump Rope	

REPEAT

CORE - 1 minute each exercise set - slow to mid-paced - 10 minutes total	
1) Cross Crunch	6) Side Planks - left
2) Floor Angel	7) Side Planks - right
3) Side to Side Crunch	8) Superman
4) Pumpers	9) Quadriped
5) Russian Twist	10) Planks

STRETCH - hold twice for 30 seconds each - slow-paced - 10 minutes total	
1) Child Pose	6) Shoulder (wall) - right
2) Cobra Pose	7) Single Shoulder/Elbow Grasp - left
3) Overhead Triceps - left	8) Single Shoulder/Elbow Grasp - right
4) Overhead Triceps - right	9) Reverse Hug
5) Shoulder (wall) - left	10) Neck ROM

First & Third Wednesday - Intervals

WARM UP - 1 minute per exercise set - mid-paced - 10 minutes total	
1) Side Bend - left	6) Trunk Rotation
2) Side Bend - right	7) Knee Up - left
3) Front & Back Bend	8) Knee Up - right
4) Helicopter	9) Stationary Jog
5) Hands Together Side Bend	10) Jumping Jacks
CARDIO - fast-paced - 5 minutes total	
1) Run/Jog ~2.5 minutes	
2) Shuttle Run (2:1 = work:rest) ~2.5 minutes	
INTERVAL TRAINING - fast-paced - 20 seconds on, 10 seconds off - 10 minutes total	
1) Jump Rope	1) Skaters
2) Calf Bounce	2) Explosive Side Lunge
3) Monkey Jacks	3) Monkey Jump
4) Soccer Tap	4) Squat Thrust
REPEAT	REPEAT
REST 1 minute after each completed circuit	
CARDIO - fast-paced- 5 minutes total	
1) Jump Rope - 40 seconds	
2) Rest - 20 seconds	
REPEAT x4	
INTERVAL TRAINING - fast-paced - 20 seconds on, 10 seconds off - 10 minutes total	
1) Mountain Climber	1) Squat Thrust
2) Knee Up - 1st set: left, 2nd set right	2) Stationary Jog
REPEAT x3	REPEAT x3
REST 1 minute after each completed circuit	
CORE - 1 minute each exercise set - slow to mid-paced - 10 minutes total	
1) Crunch	6) Pumpers
2) Bicycles	7) Side Planks - left
3) Russian Twist	8) Side Lying Leg Lift - left
4) Leg Lift	9) Side Planks - right
5) Side to Side Crunch	10) Side Lying Leg Lift - right
STRETCH - slow-paced - hold twice for 30 seconds each - 10 minutes total	
1) Standing Ankle Pick - left	6) Standing Hip Flexor - right
2) Standing Ankle Pick - right	7) Self Hug
3) Calf (wall) - left	8) Reverse Hug
4) Calf (wall) - right	9) Shoulder Roll
5) Standing Hip Flexor - left	10) Palms Interlaced Overhead

First & Third Thursday - Pull

WARM UP - 1 minute per exercise set - mid-paced - 10 minutes total	
1) Side Bend - left	6) Trunk Rotation
2) Side Bend - right	7) Knee Up - left
3) Front & Back Bend	8) Knee Up - right
4) Helicopter	9) Stationary Jog
5) Hands Together Side Bend	10) Jumping Jacks

CARDIO - fast-paced - 5 minutes total
1) Run/Jog

WEIGHT TRAINING - 1 minute per exercise - mid to fast-paced - 10 minutes total
1) DB Bent Row
2) DB Stick Up
3) DB Zottman Curl
4) DB Upright Rows & Curl
5) DB Front & Side Raise
REPEAT

CARDIO - fast-paced- 5 minutes total
1) Run/Jog

WEIGHT TRAINING - 1 minute per exercise - mid to fast-paced - 10 minutes total
1) RB Row
2) RB High Row
3) RB Curl
4) RB Trunk Rotation - left
5) RB Trunk Rotation - right
REPEAT

CORE - slow to mid-paced - 1 minute each exercise set - 10 minutes total	
1) Legs Up Crunch	6) Legs Up Cross Crunch
2) Leg Lift	7) Reverse Crunch with Leg Extension
3) Bicycle Cross Crunch	8) Russian Twist with Bicycles
4) Window Wiper	9) Flutters
5) Side to Side Crunch	10) Planks

STRETCH - slow-paced - hold twice for 30 seconds each - 10 minutes total	
1) Child Pose	6) Single Shoulder/Elbow Grasp - left
2) Overhead Triceps - left	7) Single Shoulder/Elbow Grasp - right
3) Overhead Triceps - right	8) Forearm - left
4) Reverse Hug	9) Forearm - right
5) Palms Interlaced Overhead	10) Neck ROM

First & Third Friday - Squat/Push

WARM UP - 1 minute per exercise set - mid-paced - 10 minutes total	
1) Side Bend - left	6) Trunk Rotation
2) Side Bend - right	7) Knee Up - left
3) Front & Back Bend	8) Knee Up - right
4) Helicopter	9) Stationary Jog
5) Hands Together Side Bend	10) Jumping Jacks

WEIGHT TRAINING - 1 minute per exercise - mid to fast-paced - 10 minutes	
1) Squat Thrust	
2) DB Walking Lunge	
3) DB Front & Side Raise	
4) DB Step Up - 1st set: left, 2nd set: right	
5) DB Single Leg Squat - 1st set: left, 2nd set: right	
REPEAT	

CARDIO - 20 seconds on, 10 seconds off - fast-paced- 5 minutes total	
1) Explosive Side Lunge	
2) Jumping Jacks	
3) Stationary Jog	
4) Monkey Jacks	
REPEAT, then rest 1 minute	

WEIGHT TRAINING - 1 minute per exercise - mid to fast-paced - 10 minutes	
1) DB Squat with Single Arm Cross Press - 1st set: left, 2nd set: right	
2) DB Walking Lunge with Side Raise	
3) Jump Rope	
4) DB Step Up with Arnold Press - 1st set: left, 2nd set: right	
5) DB Transverse Lunge with Stick Up - 1st set: left, 2nd set: right	
REPEAT	

CORE - 1 minute per exercise - slow to mid-paced - 10 minutes total	
1) Cross Crunch	6) Floor Angel
2) Lying Leg Extension	7) Reverse Crunch with Rotation
3) Bicycle Cross Crunch	8) Russian Twist with Bicycles
4) Scissors	9) Flutters
5) Side to Side Crunch	10) Planks

STRETCH - hold twice for 30 seconds each - slow-paced - 10 minutes total	
1) Child Pose	6) Shoulder (wall) - left
2) Kneeling Hip Flexor - left	7) Shoulder (wall) -right
3) Kneeling Hip Flexor - right	8) Forearm - left
4) Overhead Triceps - left	9) Forearm - right
5) Overhead Triceps - right	10) Neck ROM

Second & Fourth Monday - Squat

WARM UP - 1 minute per exercise set - mid-paced - 10 minutes total	
1) Side Bend - left	6) Trunk Rotation
2) Side Bend - right	7) Knee Up - left
3) Front & Back Bend	8) Knee Up - right
4) Helicopter	9) Stationary Jog
5) Hands Together Side Bend	10) Jumping Jacks

CARDIO - 30 seconds per exercise - fast-paced - 5 minutes total
1) Jump Rope
2) Pump Lunge - 1st set: left, 2nd set: right
3) Jumping Jacks
4) Jump Squat
5) Skaters
REPEAT

WEIGHT TRAINING - 1 minute per exercise - mid to fast-paced - 10 minutes total
1) Step Up with Knee Up - 1st set: left, 2nd set: right
2) Reverse Lunge with Knee Up - 1st set: left, 2nd set: right
3) Calf Raise on step
4) Squat Thrust
5) Mountain Climber
REPEAT

CARDIO - 30 seconds per exercise - fast-paced - 5 minutes total
1) Jump Rope
2) Static Squat with Heel Raise Hold
3) Forward Jacks
4) Pump Lunge - 1st set: left, 2nd set: right
5) Explosive Side Lunge
REPEAT

WEIGHT TRAINING - 1 minute per exercise - mid to fast-paced - 10 minutes total
1) DB Squat & Reverse Lunge
2) Soccer Tap
3) DB Wall Chair with Toe Tap
4) DB Pumping Sumo Squat
5) Single Leg Calf Raise - 1st set: left, 2nd set: right
REPEAT

CORE - 1 minute each exercise set - slow to mid-paced - 10 minutes total	
1) Dynamic Bridge	6) Side to Side Crunch
2) Side Lying Leg Lift - left	7) Quadriped
3) Floor Angel	8) Side Planks - left
4) Side Lying Leg Lift - right	9) Reverse Crunch with Leg Extension
5) Legs Up Cross Crunch	10) Side Planks - right

STRETCH - hold twice for 30 seconds each - slow-paced - 10 minutes total	
1) Child Pose	6) Seated Single Hamstring - right
2) Cobra Pose	7) Cross Leg Twist - left
3) Kneeling Hip Flexor - left	8) Cross Leg Twist - right
4) Kneeling Hip Flexor - right	9) Butterfly
5) Seated Single Hamstring - left	10) Knees Hug

Second & Fourth Tuesday - Pull

WARM UP - 1 minute per exercise set - mid-paced - 10 minutes total	
1) Side Bend - left	6) Trunk Rotation
2) Side Bend - right	7) Knee Up - left
3) Front & Back Bend	8) Knee Up - right
4) Helicopter	9) Stationary Jog
5) Hands Together Side Bend	10) Jumping Jacks
CARDIO - fast-paced- 5 minutes total	
1) Run/Jog	
WEIGHT TRAINING - 1 minute per exercise - mid to fast-paced - 10 minutes total	
1) DB Bent Row & Bent High Row	
2) DB Zottman Curl - alternating	
3) DB Bent Reverse Fly & Underhand Row	
4) DB Side Raise & Front Raise	
5) Soccer Tap	
REPEAT	
CARDIO - fast-paced- 5 minutes total	
1) Shuttle Run (2:1 = work:rest)	
WEIGHT TRAINING - 1 minute per exercise - mid to fast-paced - 10 minutes total	
1) RB Pulldown	
2) RB Front Pulldown	
3) RB Reverse Fly	
4) RB 21s	
5) Soccer Tap	
REPEAT	
CARDIO - fast-paced- 5 minutes total	
1) Shuttle Run (2:1 = work:rest) - 2.5 minutes	
2) Run/Jog - 2.5 minutes	
CORE - slow to mid-paced - 1 minute each exercise set - 10 minutes total	
1) Crunch	6) Jackknife
2) Reverse Crunch	7) Bicycle Cross Crunch
3) Bicycles	8) Russian Twist
4) Window Wiper	9) Cross Arm/Cross Leg Crunch
5) Legs Up Crunch	10) Planks
STRETCH - slow-paced - hold twice for 30 seconds each - 10 minutes total	
1) Child Pose	6) Single Shoulder/Elbow grasp - left
2) Cobra Pose	7) Single shoulder/Elbow grasp - right
3) Reverse Hug	8) Forearm - left
4) Straight Arm/Shoulder (wall) - left	9) Forearm - right
5) Straight Arm/Shoulder (wall) - right	10) Overhead Arm Hold (wall)

Second & Fourth Wednesday - Intervals

WARM UP - 1 minute per exercise set - mid-paced - 10 minutes total	
1) Side Bend - left	6) Trunk Rotation
2) Side Bend - right	7) Knee Up - left
3) Front & Back Bend	8) Knee Up - right
4) Helicopter	9) Stationary Jog
5) Hands Together Side Bend	10) Jumping Jacks
CARDIO - fast-paced - 5 minutes total	
1) Jump Rope - 40 seconds	
2) Static Squat - 20 seconds	
REPEAT x4	
INTERVAL TRAINING - fast-paced - 20 seconds on, 10 seconds off - 10 minutes total	
1) Monkey Jump	1) Explosive Step Up
2) Jump Lunge	2) Explosive Side Lunge
REPEAT x3	REPEAT x3
REST 1 minute after each completed circuit	
CARDIO - fast-paced- 5 minutes total	
1) Shuttle Run (2:1 = work:rest)	
INTERVAL TRAINING - fast-paced - 20 seconds on, 10 seconds off - 10 minutes total	
1) DB Jab	1) Jumping Jacks
2) DB Cross	2) Knee Up - left
3) DB Uppercut	3) Knee Up - right
4) DB Back Fist	4) Stationary Jog
REPEAT	REPEAT
REST 1 minute after each completed circuit	
CORE - slow to mid-paced - 1 minute each exercise set - 10 minutes total	
1) Cross Crunch	6) Quadriped
2) Dynamic Bridge	7) Side Planks - left
3) Wall Chair	8) Side Lying Leg Lift - left
4) Floor Angel	9) Side Planks - right
5) Planks	10) Side Lying Leg Lift - right
STRETCH - slow-paced - hold twice for 30 seconds each - 10 minutes total	
1) Kneeling Hip Flexor - left	6) Shoulder (wall) - right
2) Kneeling Hip Flexor - right	7) Standing Hip Flexor - left
3) Single Calf (pike) - left	8) Standing Hip Flexor - right
4) Single Calf (pike) - right	9) Bent Hamstring - left
5) Shoulder (wall) - left	10) Bent Hamstring - right

Second & Fourth Thursday - Push

WARM UP - 1 minute per exercise set - mid-paced - 10 minutes total	
1) Side Bend - left	6) Trunk Rotation
2) Side Bend - right	7) Knee Up - left
3) Front & Back Bend	8) Knee Up - right
4) Helicopter	9) Stationary Jog
5) Hands Together Side Bend	10) Jumping Jacks
CARDIO - fast-paced- 5 minutes total	
1) Shuttle Run (2:1 = work:rest)	
WEIGHT TRAINING - 1 minute per exercise - mid to fast-paced - 10 minutes total	
1) Push Up with Rotation	
2) DB Lying Press with Bridge	
3) DB Lying Fly with Bridge	
4) DB Lying Pullover with Bridge	
5) DB Lying French Press with Bridge	
REPEAT	
CARDIO - fast-paced- 5 minutes total	
1) Run/Jog - 60 seconds	
2) Jump Rope - 60 seconds	
3) Soccer Tap - 30 seconds	
REPEAT	
WEIGHT TRAINING -1 minute per exercise - mid to fast-paced - 10 minutes total	
1) Dip	
2) DB Front & Side Raise	
3) DB Bent Kickback	
4) DB Arnold Press	
5) DB Trunk Rotation	
REPEAT	
CORE - slow to mid-paced - 1 minute each exercise set - 10 minutes total	
1) Cross Crunch	6) Reverse Crunch with Rotation
2) Leg Lift	7) Russian Twist with Bicycle
3) Window Wiper	8) Quadriped
4) Legs Up Cross Crunch	9) Jackknife
5) Cross Arm Cross Leg Crunch	10) Planks
STRETCH - hold twice for 30 seconds each - slow-paced - 10 minutes total	
1) Child Pose	6) Shoulder (wall) - right
2) Cobra Pose	7) Single Shoulder/Elbow Grasp - left
3) Overhead Triceps - left	8) Single Shoulder/Elbow Grasp - right
4) Overhead Triceps - right	9) Reverse Hug
5) Shoulder (wall) - left	10) Neck ROM

Second & Fourth Friday - Squat/Pull

WARM UP - 1 minute per exercise set - mid-paced - 10 minutes total	
1) Side Bend - left	6) Trunk Rotation
2) Side Bend - right	7) Knee Up - left
3) Front & Back Bend	8) Knee Up - right
4) Helicopter	9) Stationary Jog
5) Hands Together Side Bend	10) Jumping Jacks

WEIGHT TRAINING - 1 minute per exercise - mid to fast-paced - 10 minutes
1) DB Squat with Curl
2) DB Reverse Lunge with Side Raise
3) DB Bent Row
4) DB Side Bend
REPEAT

CARDIO - fast-paced- 5 minutes total
1) Jump Rope - 2.5 minutes
2) Run/Jog - 2.5 minutes

WEIGHT TRAINING - 1 minute per exercise - mid to fast-paced - 10 minutes
1) RB Side Lunge with Rotation - left
2) RB Side Lunge with Rotation - right
3) RB Row with Static Squat
4) RB High Row with Static Lunge - left
5) RB Curl with Static Lunge - right
REPEAT

CARDIO - fast-paced- 5 minutes total
1) Run/Jog - 2.5 minutes
2) Shuttle Run (2:1 = work:rest) - 2.5 minutes

CORE - slow to mid-paced - 1 minute each exercise set - 10 minutes total	
1) Crunch	6) Cross Crunch
2) Reverse Crunch with Leg Extension	7) Reverse Crunch with Rotation
3) Bicycle Cross Crunch	8) Cherry Picker
4) Scissors	9) Leg Lift
5) Side to Side Crunch	10) Planks

STRETCH - hold twice for 30 seconds each - slow-paced - 10 minutes total	
1) Lying Ankle Pick - left	6) Shoulder (wall) - right
2) Lying Ankle Pick - right	7) Single Shoulder/Elbow Grasp - left
3) Single Calf (pike) - left	8) Single Shoulder/Elbow Grasp - right
4) Single Calf (pike) - right	9) Lateral Leg - left
5) Shoulder (wall) - left	10) Lateral Leg - right

Glossary of Exercises

Bent Hamstring

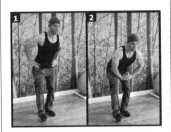

From a standing position and feet slightly separated, bring one foot further out from the other. Keep the front leg straight, bend the rear leg at the waist and knee while supporting yourself just above your knee. The further you drop your butt down, the deeper the stretch will be felt on the hamstring (back of the thigh) of the front leg. Change direction and stretch the opposite side for equal time.

Bicycle Cross Crunch with Leg Hold

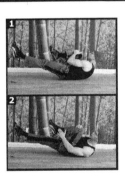

Lie on your back. Extend one leg 45° from the ground, draw the other leg into your chest and gently hug that knee while lifting the opposite shoulder. Release the hold and switch legs to repeat the movement sequence.

Helpful tip: Form, or the way you perform an exercise, isn't limited to how you move. Proper performance comes from moving correctly and breathing naturally. Without good breathing, your muscles will not perform to its fullest potential.

Bicycle Cross Crunch

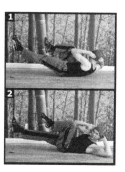

Lie flat on your back, support your head with your fingertips while keeping your elbows pulled back. Extend one leg 45° from the ground while drawing the other leg toward your chest. Simultaneously bring the opposite shoulder off the ground and drive that elbow toward the bent knee. Switch sides and repeat the movement sequence.

Bicycles

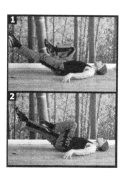

Lie flat on your back with your arms extended to your sides and palms faced down for support. Extend one leg 45° from the ground while drawing one knee toward your chest. Switch leg positions and alternate between legs for the entire exercise set.

Butterfly

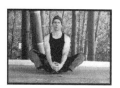

From a seated position, bend your knees and place your heels against each other. Grasp the top of your feet and draw your heels as close to your inner thigh as possible. Lift your big toes up as you press your knees down with your elbows. Keep your posture up and proud.

Calf (wall)

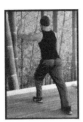

Stand facing a wall one foot away. Place your palms into the wall with your arms extended. Separate your stance about shoulder-width apart and bring one foot closer to the wall with a slight bend in that knee. The back leg should be fully extended. You should feel a good stretch in the calf area (just above the heel and below the knee) of the back leg. If a stretch is not felt, separate your feet more or step further away from the wall. Change direction and stretch the opposite side for equal time.

Calf Bounce

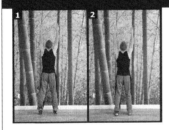

Stick your arms up, bring your feet together and raise your heels. Now, bounce rapidly on the balls of your feet.

Calf Raise on Step

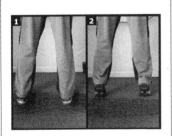

Stand on a step with your heels hanging off and the balls of your feet firmly planted. Separate your feet shoulder-width apart and raise your heels above the step, pause, then slowly return to the start position.

Calf Raise

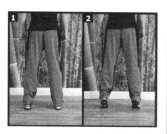

Separate your feet shoulder-width apart and raise your heels off the ground, pause, then slowly return to the ground.

Cat & Dog

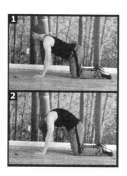

From a kneeling position and palms placed below your shoulders, arch your spine upward and look toward your knees. Then, push your spine downward and lift your chin upward.

Fun fact: The "Cat & Dog" exercise is a yoga-based movement and limbers up the spinal column. Use this exercise as a warm-up or cooldown for most any exercise routine. In fact, before you get out of bed and start your day, do "Cat & Dog" for about 3-5 minutes. It'll amaze you how much this exercise will get you feeling energetic and ready to kick ass in your day!

Cherry Picker

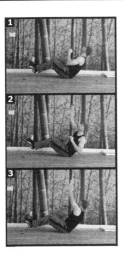

Come to a seated position on the ground with your knees bent and heels planted. Lean back onto your tailbone and reach your hands up. Reach higher with one arm then the other arm. Repeat this movement for the set.

Child Pose with Arm Thread

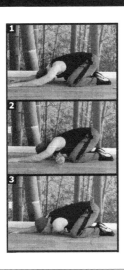

From a kneeling position, rest your butt on your heels, bend at the hips and bring your torso to rest on the ground with your arms extended above your head. Cross one extended arm in front of your chest and under the other arm. Relax and take deep breaths. Stretch the opposite side for equal time.

Child Pose

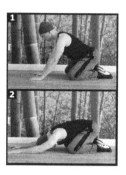

From a kneeling position, rest your butt on your heels, bend at the hips and bring your torso to rest on the ground with your arms extended above your head. Relax and take deep breaths.

Cobra Pose

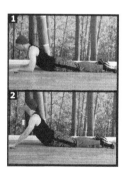

Lie on your stomach with your elbows bent below your shoulders and palms placed into the floor. Extend your arms and arch your spine upward while lifting your chin.

Helpful tip: If you sit a lot, then the "Cobra Pose" is an excellent exercise for you. Notice in the picture inset—the hips bend the opposite direction of the seated position. This stretch helps combat a lot of low back and front hip tightness.

Coffin Sit Up

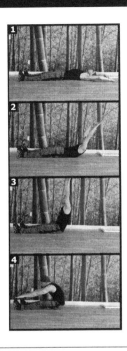

Lie on the floor with your arms by your ears, extended above your head. Slowly raise your back (one vertebra at a time) off the floor keeping your arms by your ears. When you have come to a seated position, reach toward your toes, pause, then slowly return to the start position.

Word of caution: Coffin sit-ups are not the traditional idea of momentum-driven calisthenics. You must move deliberately and pay close attention to your body mechanics. Returning to the start position is tough as hell and requires patience. The first time you try coffin sit-ups, do your best in slowly coming back down.

Cross Arm & Leg Crunch

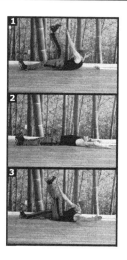

Lie on your back, completely flattened out with your arms extended above your head. Simultaneously, raise one leg and the opposite arm up to the ceiling, lift your torso up to reach your toe. Pause, then slowly return to the lying position. Repeat the movement sequence on the other side.

Cross Crunch

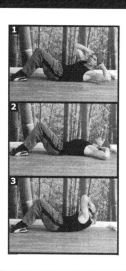

Lie on your back with your feet flat on the ground and your knees bent. Gently place your fingertips behind your head with your elbows pulled back. Slowly press one side of your ribs upward, pause at your highest position, then slowly return to the start position. Repeat the movement sequence on the other side.

Cross Leg Bridge

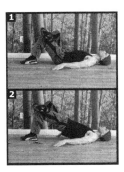

Lie on the ground with your arms out to the sides, knees bent and your feet placed flat on the floor. Cross one leg over the other with your ankle by the knee. Begin by pressing your pelvis up and hold when your torso is 45° from the floor. Pause, squeeze your butt and tighten your abs for a 3-count, then gradually lower your butt back to the ground. Repeat this movement sequence and train each side equally.

Cross Leg Twist

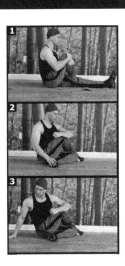

From a seated position, cross one leg over the other with your knees together. Rest your arms out to your sides with your palms on the floor. Begin to turn away from the side of the top leg and look away from the side you are twisting. Change direction and stretch the opposite side for equal time.

Helpful tip: If you are excessively rigid in your glutes (aka butt muscles), then stay in the first position of the picture inset. Hold that position until your glutes tolerate a deeper stretch.

Crunch

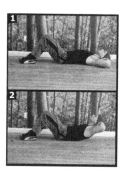

Lie flat with your back and feet flat on the ground and your knees bent. Gently place your fingertips behind your head with your elbows pulled back. Slowly press your ribs upward, pause at your highest position, then slowly return to the start position.

DB Arnold Press

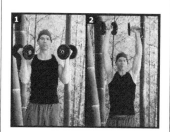

Grasp your weights at shoulder level with your elbows tucked into your ribs. Press your arms up overhead and rotate your wrists (with thumbs pointing) inward. Pause at the top, then slowly return back to the start position.

Interesting fact: Due to my history of low back injuries, my doctors discouraged me from doing any overhead exercises. These types of exercises tend to compress the spinal column and put undue pressure on the lower back. However, I lifted light weights and engaged my core with the "Stomach Flattener." The more I improved in my low back, the more weight I could handle. I'm not shattering any world records, but I improved my shoulders, midsection and low back drastically since using this modification.

DB Back Fist

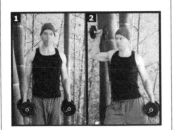

Grasp the weights at eye level with your elbows tucked in front of your chest. Draw your hands above and outside their respective shoulders with your elbows bent. Pull one elbow at a 90° outside of your shoulder with your knuckles toward the ceiling. Slowly lower your arm back to the start position. Rotate your torso toward the direction of your raised arm. Repeat the movement sequence in the other direction.

DB Bent Kickback

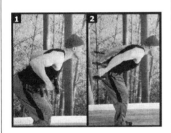

Bring your feet together, squat slightly while bending your torso at a 45° angle from the ground. Tuck your elbows up and back with your knuckles parallel with the ground. Extend your elbows, kicking your forearms back and keeping your palms faced inward. Pause and lower your forearms back until the knuckles are parallel to the ground.

WATCH OUT!—A common mistake is when you curl the dumbbells up to the shoulders. Simply extend your arm back and then bend it back toward the ground. Dumbbell kickbacks are meant for isolating the triceps. If you curl weight toward your shoulders, then you engage your biceps. There's no sense in doing unnecessary work.

Additional Tip—Keep your stomach tight as hell in this position so that you are not putting too much pressure on your low back.

DB Bent Underhand Row

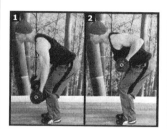

Bring your feet together, come to a slight squat with your knees bent and butt sticking out. Position your torso at about 30-45° from the ground, reach your arms toward the ground with your palms faced away from your body. Keeping your knuckles parallel to the ground at all times, pull your elbows along your ribs and toward your back. Pause at the top and slowly lower the weights back toward the ground. Keep your mid-section tight throughout the entire set.

DB Bent Reverse Fly & Overhand Row

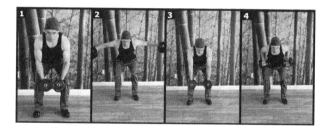

Bring your feet together, come to a slight squat with your knees bent and butt sticking out. Position your torso at about 30-45° from the ground, reach your arms toward the ground. Keeping your arms straight, separate and bring them to outside of your shoulders. Pause, then slowly lower your arms back to start position. Then, turn your palms away from your body, pull your elbows along your ribs and toward your back. Pause at the top and slowly lower the weights back toward the ground. Alternate between each movement sequence. Keep your mid-section tight throughout the entire set.

Exercise light until it's right!

DB Bent Reverse Fly

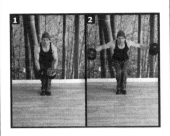

Bring your feet together, come to a slight squat with your knees bent and butt sticking out. Position your torso at about 30-45° from the ground, reach your arms toward the ground. Keeping your arms straight, separate and bring them to outside of your shoulders. Pause, then slowly lower your arms back to start position. Keep your mid-section tight throughout the entire set.

DB Bent Row & Bent High Row

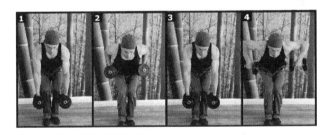

Bring your feet together, come to a slight squat with your knees bent and butt sticking out. Position your torso at about 30-45° from the ground, reach your arms toward the ground. Keeping your knuckles parallel to the ground at all times, pull your elbows along your ribs and toward your back. Pause at the top and slowly lower the weights back toward the ground. Then, angle your knuckles away from your body, pull your elbows up and away from your ribs so that your upper arms are level with your shoulders. Return to start position. Alternate between each movement sequence. Keep your mid-section tight throughout the entire set.

Helpful Tip: Keep your spine in its natural curved position when you bend for this exercise. Frequently evaluate your form.

DB Bent Row

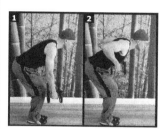

Bring your feet together, come to a slight squat with your knees bent and butt sticking out. Position your torso at about 30-45° from the ground, reach your arms toward the ground. Keeping your knuckles parallel to the ground at all times, pull your elbows along your ribs and toward your back. Pause at the top and slowly lower the weights back toward the ground. Keep your mid-section tight throughout the entire set.

DB Bent Single Arm Row

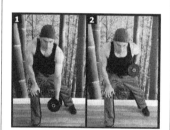

Separate your feet shoulder-width apart with your feet staggered, one further in front of the other. On the same side as your lead leg, place your free hand on your knee. Position your torso at about 30-45° from the ground, reach with your other arm with the weight toward the ground. Pull the weight bearing elbow back and up, pause, then slowly release your arm back toward the ground. After completing one side, be sure to switch your positioning and repeat the movement sequence. Keep your mid-section tight throughout the entire set.

Helpful tip: A good modification for the "Dumbbell Bent Single Arm Row" is to use a bench for support. Rather than stand, you kneel one knee on the bench while the other leg plants into the floor. People with weaker cores or anyone using heavier weights use this modification.

DB Bent Straight Arm Kickback

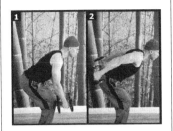

Bring your feet together, come to a slight squat with your knees bent and butt sticking out. Position your torso at about 30-45° from the ground, reach your arms toward the ground. Keep your arms parallel as you kick them back with your pinkies driving upward. Pause at the top, then slowly lower the weights to the start position. Keep your mid-section tight throughout the entire set.

DB Chicken Wing

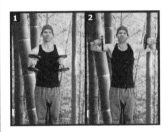

Grasp your weights with palms faced inward and elbows bent. Raise your elbows up to shoulder height, pause, then lower your elbows back to your ribs.

DB Close Foot Squat

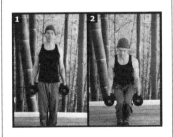

Grasp your weights at your hips with your legs together, bend your knees and butt 90° and keep your torso upright. Essentially come down to a seated position. Press through your heels, keep your big toes lifted and extend your legs back up to stand.

DB Cross

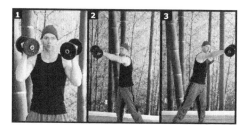

Grasp the weights at eye level with your elbows tucked in front of your chest. Extend one arm in front of the opposite shoulder, then bring it back. Alternate the movement sequence on both sides for the entire set.

DB Curl & Press

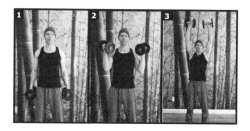

Grasp your weights with your palms faced in just outside of your hips. Slowly bend your elbows and draw your palms toward your shoulders. Press the dumbbells overhead while rotating your wrists inward. Then tuck your elbows back into your ribs, open your arms and return to the start position.

Fun Fact: People associate the "Dumbbell Arnold Press" with former-California governor, bodybuilder, and movie star, Arnold Schwarzenegger.

DB Curl

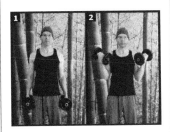

Grasp your weights with your palms face to your sides. Keep your upper arm secured snugly to your ribs. Bend at your elbows and bring your forearms toward your shoulders. As your arms come up, rotate your wrists to bring your palms to face in toward your shoulders. Slowly return back to the start position.

DB Front & Side Raise

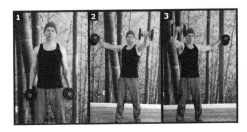

From a standing position, keep your elbows extended and arms straight for this exercise. Raise your left hand directly in front of the left shoulder while raising your right hand outside of the right shoulder. Pause, then lower the weights back to your sides. Now, raise your right hand directly in front of the right shoulder while raising your left hand outside of the left shoulder. Pause, then lower the weights back to your sides.

Funny Fact: Want to create the illusion that your soft midsection is small? Develop and build muscle in your shoulders. The wider and more tone your shoulders are, the smaller your midsection will appear.

DB Front Raise

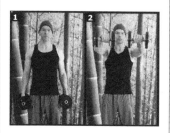

From a standing position, grasp your weights with palms faced in at your hips. Extend your arms up at shoulder level, then lower them back to start position.

DB Jab

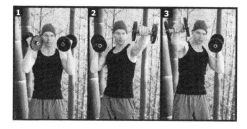

Grasp the weights at eye level with your elbows tucked in front of your chest. Extend one arm in front of the respective shoulder, then bring it back. Alternate the movement sequence on both sides for the entire set.

Words of Caution: Avoid heavy weights with "Dumbbell Jabs," because you need to control the weight as you punch forward with each movement. If you feel like the weight pulls you off balance, then you may need to decrease the amount you use.

DB Lunge

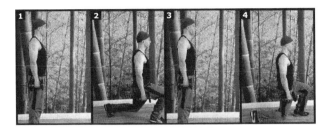

Grasp your weights at your hips and separate your feet shoulder-width apart. Step forward with one leg, bend at both knees. Pop up the rear heel and bring the knee close to the ground. Focus on a 90° bend in the front knee. Press your rear foot off the ground while driving your front heel down to bring yourself back to a standing position. Repeat the movement sequence on the other leg.

DB Lying Fly with Bridge

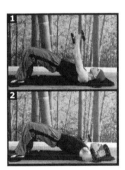

Lying on your back, pop your pelvis up, then tighten your butt and abs. Hold this position for the entirety of the exercise set. Start with your palms inward, your arms extended parallel above your sternum. Keeping your arms straight, slowly separate your arms to your sides, lowering your knuckles close to the ground. Pause, then squeeze your palms back together just above your sternum again. The bridge modification is great for core development.

Helpful tip: Master the "DB Lying Fly" before trying the "DB Lying Fly with Bridge." This exercise is for more advanced exercisers.

DB Lying Fly

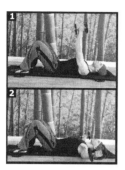

Lie on your back with your knees bent and feet flat on the floor. Start with your palms inward, your arms extended parallel above your sternum. Keeping your arms straight, slowly separate your arms to your sides, lowering your knuckles close to the ground. Pause, then squeeze your palms back together just above your sternum again.

DB Lying Press with Bridge

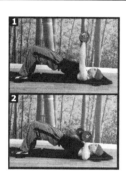

Lying on your back, pop your pelvis up, then tighten your butt and abs. Hold this position for the entirety of the exercise set. Grasp your weights with your palms face toward your feet and forearms 90° from the ground. Press your arms directly to the sky, pause when your arms are extended, then bend at the elbows and return to the start position. The bridge modification is great for core development.

Fun Fact: Why combine a bridge with a dumbbell exercise? Using a core exercise with a weighted exercise is an excellent way to integrate the whole body. And, you burn more calories when you combine an isometric exercise with a movement-based exercise.

DB Lying Press

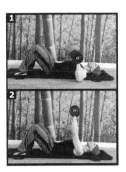

Lie on your back with your knees bent and feet flat on the ground. Grasp your weights with your palms face toward your feet and forearms 90° from the ground. Press your arms directly to the sky, pause when your arms are extended, then bend at the elbows and return to the start position.

DB Lying Pullover with Bridge

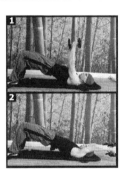

Lying on your back, pop your pelvis up, then tighten your butt and abs. Hold this position for the entirety of the exercise set. Start with your palms faced inward, your arms extended parallel above your sternum. Keeping your arms straight, slowly lower your arms above your head. When your biceps become flush with your ears, pause, then drive your arms back to the start position. This modification is great for core development.

Fun Fact: The "Dumbbell Pullover" is a multi-purpose exercise that primarily works the back and chest. Have you ever noticed fitness models with the muscle ridge along the ribs and right below the armpits? That area is called the serratus anterior. Pullovers target the serratus anterior and help give it a defined look.

DB Lying Pullover

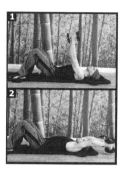

Lie on your back with your knees bent and feet flat on the ground. Start with your palms faced inward, your arms extended parallel above your sternum. Keeping your arms straight, slowly lower your arms above your head. When your biceps become flush with your ears, pause, then drive your arms back to the start position.

DB Overhead Extension

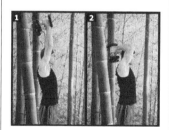

From a standing position, keep your arms parallel for this exercise. Extend your arms overhead with your palms faced inward. Bend your elbows 90°, so that the dumbbells almost touch the back of your shoulders. Pause, then slowly extend your arms back to overhead.

DB Overhead Press

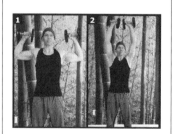

Grasp your weights at ear level with your elbows and armpit each at 90°. Press your arms overhead to meet in the middle. Slowly lower your weights back to ear level.

DB Overhead Pull with Extension

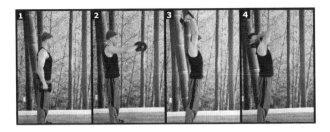

Grasp your weights at your sides with your palms faced inward. Keep your arms straight and pull the weights forward to overhead. Pause, then bend at the elbows allowing the weights to go downward behind you. Extend your elbows, driving the weights upward, then gradually allow the straightened arms to return to the start position.

DB Overhead Pull

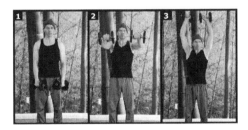

Grasp your weights at your sides with your palms faced inward. Keep your arms straight and pull the weights directly forward then up overhead. Pause, then gradually allow the straightened arms to return to the start position.

Helpful Tip: Start the "Dumbbell Overhead Pull" with light weights and gradually increase the weight over a 90-day period—no more than 5 pounds at a time.

DB Pumping Sumo Squat

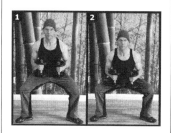

Separate your feet wider than shoulder-width apart with your toes pointed outward and weights grasped at your mid-section. Bend at the knees and lower your butt as far as possible. Slightly squat up and down, and rapidly repeat this movement sequence for the entire exercise set.

DB Reverse Lunge with Side Raise & Trunk Rotation

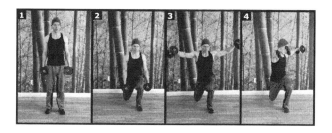

Separate your feet shoulder-width apart and grasp your weights at your hips. Step back with one leg, bend at both knees. Pop up the rear heel and bring the knee close to the ground. Focus on a 90° bend in the front knee. Raise your straightened arms with knuckles up to shoulder level. Rotate your torso toward your lead leg, return to the forward position. Pause, then lower the weights back to your sides. Press your rear foot off the ground while driving your front heel down to bring yourself back to a standing position.

*Words of Caution: The "Dumbbell Reverse Lunge with Side Raise & Trunk Rotation" is hard to say and **way** harder to do. This exercise is only intended for advanced exercisers.*

DB Reverse Lunge with Side Raise

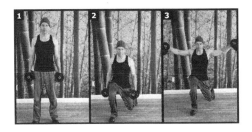

Separate your feet shoulder-width apart and grasp your weights at your hips. Step back with one leg, bend at both knees. Pop up the rear heel and bring the knee close to the ground. Focus on a 90° bend in the front knee. Raise your straightened arms with knuckles up to shoulder level. Pause, then lower the weights back to your sides. Press your rear foot off the ground while driving your front heel down to bring yourself back to a standing position.

DB Reverse Lunge

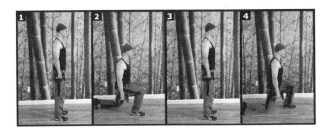

Grasp your weights at your hips and separate your feet shoulder-width apart. Step back with one leg, bend at both knees. Pop up the rear heel and bring the knee close to the ground. Focus on a 90° bend in the front knee. Press your rear foot off the ground while driving your front heel down to bring yourself back to a standing position. Repeat the movement sequence on the other leg.

DB Side Lunge with Knee Up

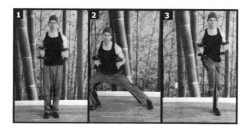

Start with your feet together and weights grasped at your hips. Step one foot to the side while keeping the other leg straight, squat down on the lead leg at a 90° bend in the hip and knee. Press off on the heel of your lead leg and come back to the start position. As you come to a standing position, bring the rear knee up in front of your hip. Repeat the movement sequence without pausing. Repeat this movement sequence and train each side equally.

DB Side Raise

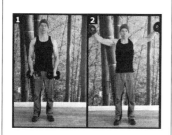

Grasp your weights at your sides. Raise your straightened arms with knuckles up to shoulder level. Pause, then lower the weights back to your sides.

Biased Note: The "Dumbbell Side Raise" is one of the most effective exercises for building size on the lateral deltoids (the side of the shoulders). Master this exercise and you will build quality muscle. Start light, go slow, pause at the top and go down even slower.

DB Single Leg Calf Raise

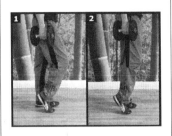 Grasp your weights at your hips, raise one heel and keep your toes placed into the ground. Bear all your weight on the flat foot. Press the flat heel upward, pause at the top, then lower your heel toward the ground. Train each side equally.

DB Single Leg Squat with Curl

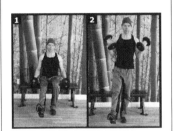 Sit down on a bench, extend one leg out in front of you and grasp your weights at your hips. Drive your other heel into the ground and stand up on that leg. Once you are fully standing, bend your elbows and turn your palms up toward your shoulders. Return your arms to your sides, then slowly squat down on the same leg until you are seated again. If balance is an issue, keep your place the heel of your extended leg into the ground. After one set, switch sides to train equally.

Words of Caution: Master the "Single Leg Squat" without dumbbells before you try the exercise with weights. Most people find balance difficult in this exercise, so you'll want to keep your hands free to catch your balance sometimes. Once you comfortably squat, add the dumbbells to the routine. Then, you may add curls to the exercise.

DB Single Leg Squat

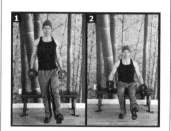

Sit down on a bench, extend one leg out in front of you and grasp your weights at your hips. Drive your other heel into the ground and stand up on that leg. Then slowly squat down on the same leg until you are seated again. If balance is an issue, keep your place the heel of your extended leg into the ground. After one set, switch sides to train equally.

DB Sit Down

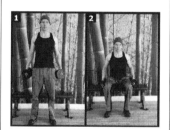

Grasp your weights at your sides and sit down. Now stand up. Focus on leading with your butt into the seat and keeping your torso upright. Sit gently. Dig your heels into the ground and press your legs back up to a standing position. Repeat this movement sequence rapidly.

Beginner's Tip: You can't squat? Then try the "Sit Down" without dumbbells. This exercise is great for training your legs while protecting your knees and back. Follow the same cues as a regular squat, but use the safety net of the chair/bench.

Watch Out!—When you stand up, don't lean your body forward and press of on your toes. This incorrect form puts undue pressure on your knees and low back.

DB Squat & Lunge

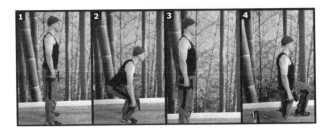

Grasp your weights at your hips with your legs shoulder-width apart. Bend your knees and butt 90° and keep your torso upright. Essentially come down to a seated position. Press through your heels, keep your big toes lifted and extend your legs back up to stand. Then, step forward with one leg, bend at both knees. Pop up the rear heel and bring the knee close to the ground. Focus on a 90° bend in the front knee. Press your rear foot off the ground while driving your front heel down to bring yourself back to a standing position. Alternate between each movement sequence and train each leg equally.

Helpful Tip:
Anytime an exercise has multiple movements in the title, assume that it is an advanced option. If you are new to exercising, split up your time with equal training time on each movement.

As an example, the "Dumbbell Squat & Lunge" separates into:
30 seconds – Dumbbell Squats
30 seconds – Dumbbell Lunges

DB Squat & Reverse Lunge

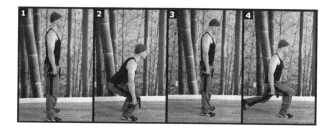

Grasp your weights at your hips with your legs shoulder-width apart. Bend your knees and butt 90° and keep your torso upright. Essentially come down to a seated position. Press through your heels, keep your big toes lifted and extend your legs back up to stand. Then, step back with one leg, bend at both knees. Pop up the rear heel and bring the knee close to the ground. Focus on a 90° bend in the front knee. Press your rear foot off the ground while driving your front heel down to bring yourself back to a standing position. Alternate between each movement sequence and train each leg equally.

DB Squat with Curl & Press

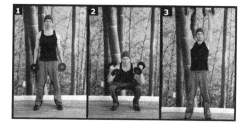

Separate your legs shoulder-width apart and keep your weights at your hips. Bend your knees and butt at 90° and keep your torso upright. As you squat down, bend your elbows and draw your palms toward your shoulders. Simultaneously, stand up and press the dumbbells overhead while rotating your wrists inward. Then tuck your elbows back into your ribs, open your arms and return to them to your hips.

DB Squat with Curl

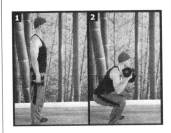

Separate your legs shoulder-width apart and your weights at your hips. Bend your knees and butt at 90° and keep your torso upright. When you are squatted down, bend your elbows and draw your palms toward your shoulders. Open your arms and return them to your hips. Press through the heels, keep your big toes lifted and extend your legs back up to stand.

DB Squat with Single Arm Cross Press

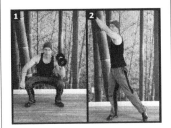

Separate your legs shoulder-width apart and keep your weights at your shoulders with your elbows bent (in a curl position). Bend your knees and butt at 90° and keep your torso upright. Press through the heels, keep your big toes lifted and extend your legs back up to stand. At the same time press one arm across your body and overhead. Load the weight up into the curl position as you squat down again.

Helpful Tip: For an aerobic burn, try the "Dumbbell Squat with Single Arm Cross Press" with a light weight. Then, perform the exercise rapidly. Your heart rate will increase in no time and you will be sweating like hell in no time!

DB Squat

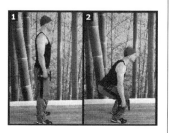

Grasp your weights at your hips with your legs shoulder-width apart. Bend your knees and butt 90° and keep your torso upright. Essentially come down to a seated position. Press through your heels, keep your big toes lifted and extend your legs back up to stand.

DB Squatted Concentration Curl

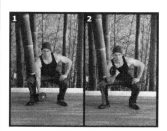

Separate your legs shoulder-width apart, bend your knees and butt at 90° and keep your torso upright. Hold the squat and brace with one hand placed on your knee. Place the outside of one elbow into the inside middle of your thigh. Bend at the elbow and bring your palm up to your shoulder, pause, then return your arm toward the ground.

DB Standing Preacher Curl

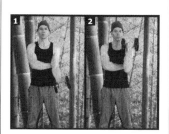

From a standing position, grasp one dumbbell in your hand with your palm faced away from your body. With your free hand, grip your ribs on your opposite side just above the back of your weight bearing elbow. Bend your elbow and curl the weight up toward your shoulder. Gradually allow your arm to open up, stopping just short of full extension.

DB Step Up with Arnold Press

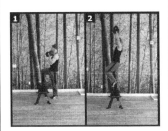

Grasp your weights at shoulder level with your elbows tucked into your ribs. Place one foot on a bench and drive your weight through that heel to bring yourself to a standing position on the bench. Simultaneously press your arms up overhead and rotate your wrists (with thumbs pointing) inward. At the same time as you start to step up, press off with the toes of your foot on the ground. When you have come to a full standing position on the bench, slowly lower the foot that pressed off the ground and bring your arms back to the start position. Repeat the movement sequence on the other leg to train equally.

DB Step Up

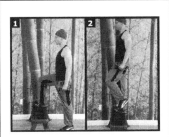

Grasp your weights at your hips. Place one foot on a bench and drive your weight through that heel to bring yourself to a standing position on the bench. At the same time as you start to step up, press off with the toes of your foot on the ground. When you have come to a full standing position on the bench, slowly lower the foot that pressed off the ground, then bring the driver leg to the ground. Repeat the movement sequence on the other leg to train equally.

Beginner's Tip: With the "Step Up," start on a low level and hold no weights.

DB Stick Up

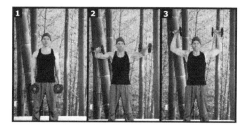

From a standing position, load your arms in front with your palms faced toward your hips. Draw your hands above and outside the respective shoulders with your elbows bent. Focus on pulling your knuckles and elbows together toward your back. Lower your arms back to the start position.

DB Sumo Squat with Curl & Press

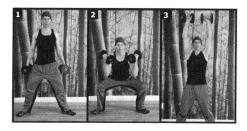

Separate your feet wider than shoulder-width apart with your toes angled outward. Grasp a weight in each hand at hip level and palms faced away from the body. Squat down to a seated position while simultaneously bending the elbows to bring the palms to the shoulders. Squat up and press the dumbbells upward while rotating the wrists so that the thumbs turn inward. Bring the dumbbells back down, guiding your elbows to your ribs as you rotate the wrists outward, then open the arms up, returning your hands back to your hips.

DB Sumo Squat

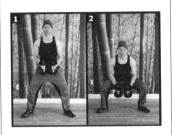

Grasp your weights at your hips and separate your feet wider than shoulder-width apart with your toes pointed outward. Bend at the knees and lower your butt as far as possible. Pause, then press through your heels and stand back up.

DB Transverse Lunge with Stick Up

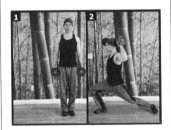

Start with your feet together and your weights grasped in front of your hips. Step one foot directly out to the side and turn your torso and toe outward before planting the foot. While keeping the other leg straight, squat down on the lead leg with a 90° bend in the hip and knee. Draw your hands above and outside the respective shoulders with your elbows bent. Focus on pulling your knuckles and elbows together toward your back. Lower your arms back to the start position, then press off on the heel of your lead leg to come back to the start position.

Helpful Tip: Master the "Transverse Lunge" without weights before you progress to the weighted variations.

Beginner's Tip: Use no weights until you master "Transverse Lunges" and "Dumbbell Stick Ups" individually.

DB Transverse Lunge

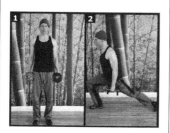

Grasp your weights at your hips and start with your feet together. Step one foot directly out to the side and turn your torso and toe outward before planting the foot. While keeping the other leg straight, squat down on the lead leg with a 90° bend in the hip and knee. Press off on the heel of your lead leg and come back to the start position.

DB Trunk Rotation

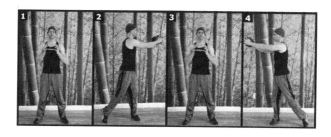

Grasp your weight in both hands in front of your sternum. Separate your feet shoulder-width apart and rotate your body to one direction. As you are rotating, extend your arms out toward that direction, then come back to the starting position. Repeat the movement sequence in the other direction.

Fun Fact: Anytime you do an exercise involving rotation at the trunk, you train your core area—primarily the obliques or side of your abs. Perform rotational movements slow and squeeze at the furthest point of a movement for better results.

DB Uppercut

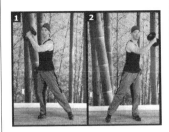

Separate your feet shoulder-width apart. Grasp a weight in each hand with your palms faced up, elbows bent slightly. In an upward arching-fashion, drive your hand with knuckles up in front of the opposite side. Pop your heel up that you are turning away form while pivoting on your body toward the direction of the uppercut. Repeat the movement sequence on the other side.

DB Upright Row & Curl

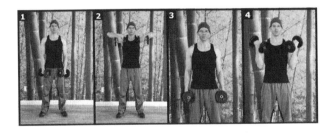

Grasp your weights with your palms faced in at your hips. Draw your elbows up to shoulder level, then return your weights to your sides. Bend at your elbows and bring your forearms toward your shoulders. As your arms come up, rotate your wrists to bring your palms to face in toward your shoulders. Slowly return back to the start position. Alternate between the movement sequences for the entire exercise set.

Words of Encouragement: If you are new to exercising, it can be discouraging seeing so many exercises. Learn one exercise per day and don't move onto the next one till you've committed it to memory.

DB Upright Row

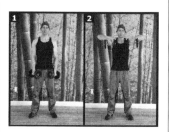

Grasp your weights with your palms faced in at your hips. Draw your elbows up to shoulder level. Then return to the start position.

DB Walking Lunge with Side Raise and Trunk Rotation

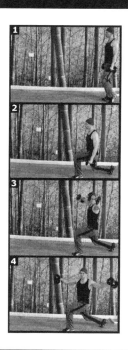

Grasp your weights at your hips and separate your feet shoulder-width apart. Step forward with one leg, bend at both knees. Pop up the rear heel and bring the knee close to the ground. Focus on a 90° bend in the front knee. Raise your straightened arms with knuckles up to shoulder level. Rotate your torso toward your lead leg, return to the forward position. Pause, then lower the weights back to your sides. Press your rear foot off the ground while driving your front heel down to bring yourself back to a standing position. Immediately bring the rear foot forward and begin the movement sequence on the other leg.

DB Walking Lunge with Side Raise

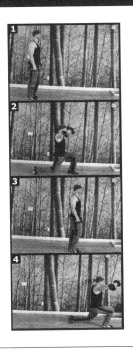

Separate your feet shoulder-width apart and grasp your weights with your palms faced in at your hips. Step forward with one leg, bend at both knees. Pop up the rear heel and bring the nee close to the ground. Primarily focus on a 90° bend in the front knee. Pause, raise your straightened arms outside of your shoulders, then lower them back down to your hips. Press your rear foot off the ground while driving your front heel down to bring yourself back to a standing position. Immediately bring your rear forward and begin the sequence on that side now, essentially performing a walking-like lunge.

Helpful Tip/Fun Fact: Many people assume that "Forward Lunges" are the simplest form of the lunge exercise. However, the easiest way to start lunging is by using the "Walking Lunge" first. The forward momentum makes it easier to handle versus stepping forward and then pushing back.

Before you use "Forward Lunges," try using "Walking Lunges." As usual, try the exercise without the weights first.

DB Walking Lunge

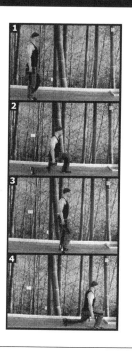

Grasp your weights at your hips and separate your feet shoulder-width apart. Step forward with one leg, bend at both knees. Pop up the rear heel and bring the knee close to the ground. Focus on a 90° bend in the front knee. Press your rear foot off the ground while driving your front heel down to bring yourself back to a standing position. Immediately bring the rear foot forward and begin the movement sequence on the other leg.

Personal Insight: My wife and I travel quite a bit and sometimes don't have the luxury of a gym. We love to challenge ourselves will often use one bodyweight exercise for an extreme number of repetitions.

Bored on time at our hotel, we decided to do walking lunges around the entire hotel parking lot. We completed a total of 1500 repetitions! I was excessively sore for days afterward, whew! Don't try this at home.

DB Zottman Curl

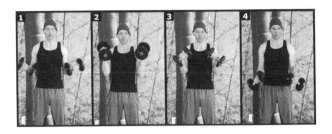

Start with your arms at your sides while grasping your weights with your palms forward. Keep your upper arm secured snugly at your ribs throughout the movement. Bend at the elbow and bring the weights toward your shoulders. The closer you come to our shoulders, the more you rotate your wrist to point your thumbs inward. Once you've reached your shoulders, your palms should be faced down. Avoid pausing and begin dropping your arms back to the start position. The closer you get to your hips, the more you rotate your thumbs back out. Make it one fluid motion up and down.

Dip

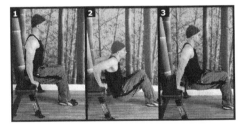

Sit down and grasp the edge of the bench. Walk your legs out and slide your butt off the bench while keeping your torso upright and arms straight. Bend at your elbows, allowing your butt to lower to the ground. Stop when your elbows are at 90°, pause, press up and extend your elbows back to the start position.

Dynamic Bridge with Heel Raise

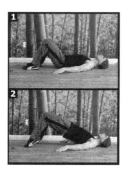

Lie on the ground with your arms out to the sides, knees bent and your feet placed flat on the floor. Press your pelvis up and hold when your torso is 45° from the floor. Raise your heels, squeeze your butt and tighten your abs for a 3-count, then gradually lower your heels and butt back to the ground. Repeat this movement sequence.

Dynamic Bridge

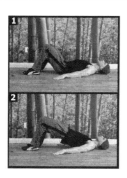

Lie on the ground with your arms out to the sides, knees bent and your feet placed flat on the floor. Press your pelvis up and hold when your torso is 45° from the floor. Raise your heels, squeeze your butt and tighten your abs for a 3-count, then gradually lower your heels and butt back to the ground. Repeat this movement sequence.

Fun Fact: The bridge is one of the most effective exercises for overall core development. You will find this exercise throughout many of my publications, blogs, and emails.

As a challenge, hold the bridge for 30-60 seconds at a time.

Explosive Side Lunge

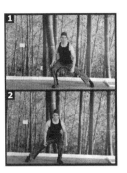

Step one leg straight to the side while bending 90° at the hip and knee. Explode up and switch legs. Rapidly repeat this movement sequence.

Explosive Step Up

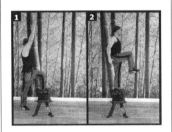

Place one foot on a bench and drive your weight through that heel to bring yourself to a standing position on the bench. Explosively press off with the toes of your foot on the ground and drive your leg to burst slightly off the bench. Without rest return to the ground, then bring the driver leg to the ground. Alternate legs for the movement sequence.

Fun Fact: The explosive movements are commonly known as plyometrics or jump training. These are exercises where you muscle exerts the maximum force for short intervals of time to increase power, speed, and strength.

Figure-4

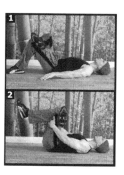

Lie on your back, cross one leg over the other with the ankle by the knee. Grasp the bottom thigh and draw it toward your chest. Stretch the opposite side for equal time.

Floor Angel

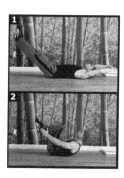

Lie on your back with your legs extended 45° from the ground and your arms raised above your head. Raise your upper body up as your draw your knees back toward your chest. Simultaneously sweep your arms outward and down to touch your ankles when the legs have come to meet the chest. Return to the start position.

Personal Insight: I may owe royalties to one of my clients for coining the name "Floor Angels." He named the exercise after making snow angels on the ground. I used to call them "Reverse Crunches with Heel Tap."

Flutter

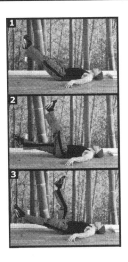

Lie on your back with your arms extended out to the side and palms faced down. Draw your legs together and up 45° from the floor (or higher for decreased difficulty). Move one leg higher than the other and alternate positions. Keep performing this sequence slow and steady while keeping your low back flat on the floor.

Forearm

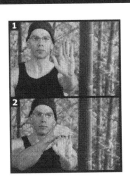

Extend one arm in front of your shoulder with your palm faced away from your body and fingers pointed up. Grasp your fingertips with your free hand and pull back. Stretch the opposite side for equal time.

Helpful Tip: The "Forearm" stretch is an excellent exercise if you spend a lot of time typing. I frequently use this stretch when I'm writing my books or working out my upper body.

Forward Jack

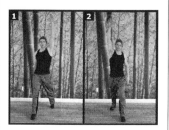

Jump up and stagger your feet with one foot further in front of the other. Keep your hand down on the side of the lead leg and raise the hand up on the rear leg. Rapidly repeat this movement sequence.

Front & Back Bend

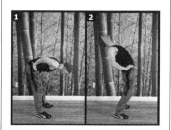

From a standing position, place your hands on your hips. Bend at the waist as far forward as you can go. Pause, squeeze your abs for a 3-count, then come back up. Without stopping, bend back as far as you can go, then immediately return to the start position.

Fun Fact: Did you know that most exercises double as strength training and flexibility training? This means that you build and stretch your muscle at the same time. These type of exercises are called dynamic stretching. The "Front & Back Bend" is a prime example of dynamic stretching.

Hands Together Side Bend

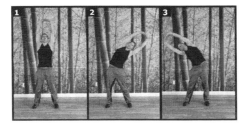

From a standing position, extend your arms overhead, interlace your fingers together and turn your palms upward with your biceps by your ears. Bend to one side as far as you can go and hold for a 5-count. Tighten your mid-section and bring yourself back to the start position. Repeat the movement sequence on the other side.

Helicopter

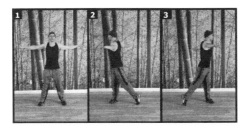

From a standing position, separate your feet shoulder-width apart and extend your arms directly outside your shoulders. Rotate at your torso, pop up the heel you are turn away from and pivot on the ball of that foot. When you have reached the farthest point, squeeze your abs, then return to the start position. Repeat the movement sequence in the other direction.

Fun Fact: Abs are made in the kitchen, not the gym.

Hip Thrust

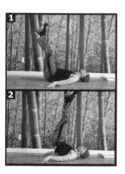

Lie on your back with your arms extended with palms faced down to aid in balance. Extend your legs toward the ceiling. Lift your butt and press your feet toward the ceiling, pause, then gradually lower yourself.

Jackknife

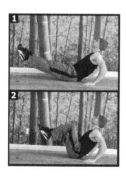

Come to a seated position on the ground with your knees bent and heels planted. Lean back onto your tailbone, extend your arms behind you with your palms placed into the ground for support. Extend your legs straight out, then draw your knees back in toward your chest. Repeat this movement sequence for the exercise set.

Helpful Tip: You can do the "Jackknife" exercise on the end of a bench. This way, you extend your legs at a lower angle for more difficulty.

Jump Squat

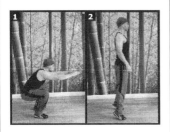

Separate your feet shoulder-width apart. Squat with your butt toward the ground, bending your hips and knees at a 90° angle. When your body has come to a near seated position, explode upwards with your legs straightened out. Shoot for jumping as high as possible and carefully landing feet first onto the ground.

Jumping Jack

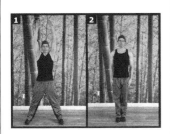

Start from a standing position, feet together and arms at your sides. In one explosive movement, jump up, separate your feet shoulder width apart while rotating your arms widely from your side to overhead. Without pause, jump again and return to the start position.

Jumping Lunge

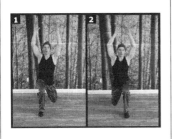

Separate your feet shoulder-width apart and step forward with one foot. Pop your rear heel up as you bend at both knees. When your lead knee comes to a 90° bend and the rear knee comes close to the ground, explode up and bring your rear leg forward and your lead leg back. Repeat the movement sequence, switching sides every jump.

Knee Hug

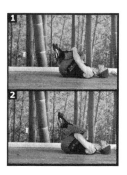

Lie on your back, draw your knees into your chest and hug them.

Knee Up

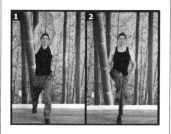

From a standing position, stagger your stance with your weight placed on the lead leg and the back heel raised. Draw your hands directly overhead and rapidly bring them down while bringing your rear knee up to meet in the middle. Quickly return to start position.

Helpful Tip: Don't like an exercise in your home workout plan? Then, exchange it for a comparable exercise so that you enjoy your workout, not dread it. You shouldn't have to tolerate working out. Embrace and relish the opportunity to exercise!

Kneeling Hip Flexor

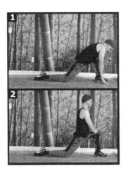

From a kneeling position, bring one leg forward, bend at the knee and place your foot flat. Place both hands on your knees and draw your posture upright. To deepen the stretch bring your foot further forward as you leave your kneeling leg in place. Stretch the opposite side for equal time.

Lateral Leg

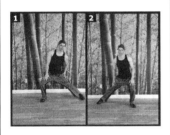

Separate your stance as wide as possible. Bend one leg at 90° in the hip and knee while keeping your upper body upright. The more you lean toward your straightened leg, the deeper the stretch is felt. Stretch the opposite side for equal time.

Helpful Tip: Stretches are best used after a workout rather than before. No peer-reviewed scientific data has proven the effectiveness of stretching for a warm-up or reducing injury. But, everyone agrees that stretching feels great for relieving tightness and muscle soreness directly after a workout.

Leg Lift

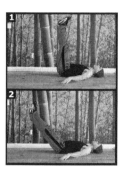

Lie on your back and extend your legs together 45° from the ground. Slowly raise your legs to point upward, then lower your legs to the start position. Repeat the movement sequence for the entire exercise set.

Legs Up Cross Crunch

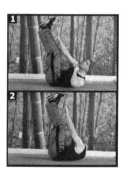

Lie on your back, extend your legs up and hold. Place your hands together, then slowly crunch up to reach one foot, pause at your highest position, then slowly return to the start position. Repeat this movement sequence in the other direction.

Helpful Tip: If you find that any variation of a lying leg lift is difficult, then raise your legs higher up. If you need more of a challenge, then lower your extended legs closer to the ground.

CAUTION: Try to keep your low back pressed into the floor to ensure safety.

Legs Up Crunch

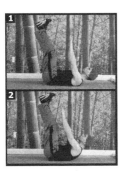

Lie on your back, extend your legs up and hold. Place your hands together, then slowly crunch up to reach your toes, pause at your highest position, then slowly return to the start position.

Lying Ankle Pick

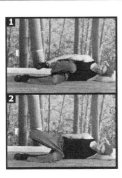

Lie on your side, draw your bottom knee up to hip level and grasp the top ankle. Pull your top heel back to your butt and hold. Stretch the opposite side for equal time.

Lying Leg Extension Hold

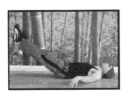

Lie on your back, extend one leg to the ceiling with the other relaxed on the ground. Grasp your extended leg at your thigh and guide it back (keeping your knee straight). Stretch the opposite side for equal time.

Lying Leg Extension

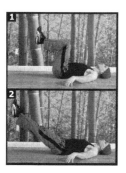

Lie on your back with your arms placed out to your sides and your palms down. Bend your hips, knees and ankles at 90° so that your lower legs are parallel with the ground and your low back is kept flat on the floor. Extend your legs out at 45° from the ground. Draw your legs back to the start position.

Monkey Jack

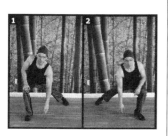

Separate your feet shoulder-width apart and stagger one foot further in front of the other. Bend slightly at the waist and reach to the ground with the arm opposite the lead leg. Jump upward, switch your feet from front to back and reach to the ground with the other arm. Rapidly repeat this movement sequence.

Monkey Jump

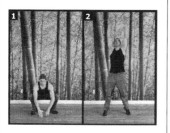

Separate your stance a little wider than shoulder-width apart with your toe turned slightly out. Reach your hands toward the ground between your legs. Immediately explode up and reach for the sky. As you land, squat deeply and reach for the ground. Rapidly repeat this movement sequence.

Mountain Climber

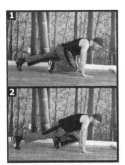

Begin with your palms placed shoulder-width apart flat on the floor and your body straight with your toes placed into the floor. You should be straight from ankles to shoulders and your vision directed at the floor between your palms. Bounce your feet slightly off the ground, drive one knee up toward the chest, and land both feet into the ground. Again, bounce your feet up, extend your forward leg back while driving your other knee up toward the chest and land both feet in the ground. Your mid-section should remain tight and rigid and avoid collapsing or extending at your hips while keeping your spinal alignment neutral throughout the movement. Repeat this movement sequence.

Neck ROM (range-of-motion)

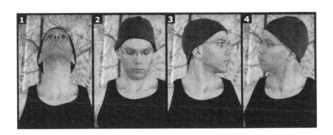

Look up and raise your chin up as high as you can and hold. Look down and drive the crown of your head as high as you can and hold. Bring your head back to neutral. Turn your chin left and hold. Then turn to the right and hold.

Overhead Interlaced Palms

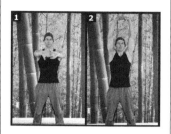

Interlace your palms, then extend your arms overhead and rotate your interlaced palms upward.

Overhead Arm Hold (wall)

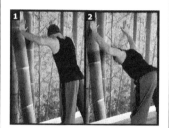

Face toward a wall within arms-reach. Extend your arms overhead and place your palms into the wall. Bend at the waist while keeping your arms above you.

Personal Insight: Isn't it funny that some of the simplest movements in this book, you probably knew all along? Sometimes, fitness requires a gentle reminder to get you going in the right direction. Come back to this book later and read through a few exercises to jog your memory. I revisit my favorite fitness books (not mine, of course) to reinvigorate my workout routine.

Overhead Triceps

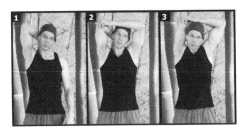

Reach one arm overhead, bend that elbow and touch the back of your neck. With your free hand, grasp your elbow overhead, guide it back and allow your hand to slide down to your back. Stretch the opposite side for equal time.

Planks with Leg Lift

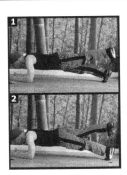

Begin with your legs separated shoulder-width apart and your toes placed into the ground for support. Place your forearms flat on the floor with your elbows bent at 90°. You should be straight from ankles to shoulders and keep your head at a neutral position with your eye sight set on your hands. As you hold your position, tighten your abs and butt. Then, lift one leg off the floor while holding your position steady. Alternate leg lift throughout the entire exercise set.

Helpful Tips: Try to perform the "Planks" exercise for 30 seconds without any movement before trying it with leg lifts. This exercise can be a lot of fun if you do it with a workout partner. Pass a ball or weight back and forth for a challenging variation.

Planks

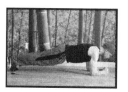

Begin with your legs separated shoulder-width apart and your toes placed into the ground for support. Place your forearms flat on the floor with your elbows bent at 90°. You should be straight from ankles to shoulders and keep your head at a neutral position with your eye sight set on your hands. As you hold your position, tighten your abs and butt.

Pop Squat

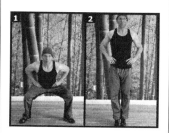

Begin in a squatted position with your legs separated shoulder-width apart, knees and butt bent at a 90° angle and torso upright. Explode up, straighten your legs and bring your feet to tap together on the ground. Then, lift both feet back up, bend your legs and return to the squat. The tap in the middle should be brief and the movement rapid.

Pump Lunge

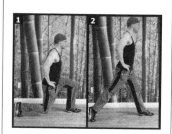

Separate your feet shoulder-width apart and place your hands on your hips. Step forward with one leg, bend at both knees. Pop up the rear heel and bring the knee close to the ground. Focus on a 90° bend in the front knee. Keep your feet in the same position and straighten both legs to staggered standing position. Repeat the movement sequence for a timed set. Train both side equally.

Pumper

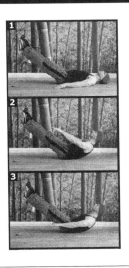

Lie on your back with your arms extended out to the side and palms faced down. Draw your legs together and up 45° from the floor (or higher for decreased difficulty) and lift your ribs up keeping your spine erect. Extend your arms along your sides parallel to the ground, then slowly pump them up and down for a timed set.

Push Up - bench - close grip

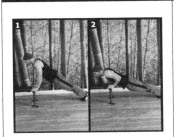

Place your palms together into the bench with your arms straight. Place your feet a few feet away from the bench. Keep your body rigid from your feet to your shoulders throughout the movement. Bend the elbows 90°, pause, then push back up, extending at the elbows.

Helpful Tip: If push-ups are too difficult for you, then try to do them against the wall with your feet about 3-4 feet away from the baseboard. Though it is simpler, it can be effective.

Push Up - bench

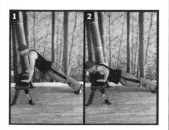

Place your palms into the bench below your shoulders with your arms straight. Place your feet a few feet away from the bench. Keep your body rigid from your feet to your shoulders throughout the movement. Bend the elbows 90°, pause, then push back up, extending at the elbows.

Push Up - staggered

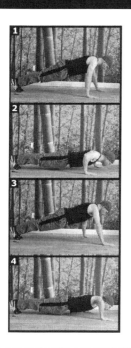

Place your palms into the ground with one hand 2-3 inches above the other and arms straightened. Keep your body rigid from your feet to your shoulders throughout the movement. Bend 90°, pause, then push yourself back up, extending at the elbows. Equally train opposite hand positions.

What seems impossible today will one day become your warm-up.

Push Up Planks

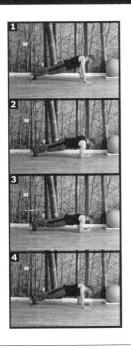

Place our palms into the ground below your shoulders with your arms straight. Keep your body rigid from your feet to your shoulders throughout the movement. Bend one elbow and place that forearm on the ground, then bend the other elbow and place the other forearm into the ground. Extend one arm and place the palm into the ground, then repeat with the other arm. Repeat the movement sequence rapidly.

Helpful Tip: Pace yourself when doing "Push Up Planks" because this exercise will tire you out in no time if you aren't careful. If it is too difficult for you to do, place your arms on a bench. In the event that is still too hard, try using the wall for this exercise.

As with any isometric exercise, breathe naturally and take your time coming to your feet afterward.

Push Up with Rotation

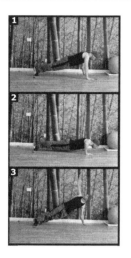

Place your palms into the ground below your shoulders with your arms straight. Keep your body rigid from your feet to your shoulders throughout the movement. Bend at the elbows 90°, pause, then push yourself back up, extending at the elbows. As your arms come to full extension, begin to lift one arm up and rotate your pelvis perpendicular to the floor. At the top position your hand should be pointed upward. Pause, then slowly lower yourself back to the start position. Repeat the movement sequence in the other direction on the subsequent repetition.

Push Up

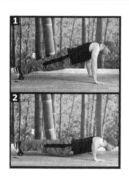

Place your palms into the ground below your shoulders with your arms straight. Keep your body rigid from your feet to your shoulders throughout the movement. Bend 90°, pause, then push back up, extending at the elbows.

"How many push-ups do you do? I don't know. I only start counting when it starts hurting.
-Muhammad Ali

Quadruped

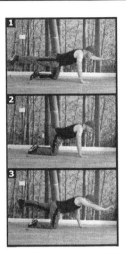

Come to a kneeling position, bend at the hips 90°, then place your hands below your shoulders with your arms extended. Raise one arm and the opposite leg parallel to the floor. Squeeze the butt and tighten the abs for a 3-count, then slowly lower back down. Repeat the movement sequence on the opposite side.

RB 21s

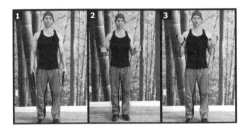

Step on the rubber band with one foot (easy difficulty) or both feet (hard difficulty). Grasping the band at hip level, secure your elbows by your ribs and stand up straight. Bend the elbows and bring your palms up toward your shoulders, pause when your forearms are parallel with the ground, then return to the start. Repeat this 7 times. Then, start with your forearms parallel with the ground and curl up to the shoulders, pause, then release to this start position. Perform this movement sequence 7 times. Lastly, bend at the elbows and bring your palms up to your shoulders, pause, then gradually return to your hips. Perform this last movement sequence 7 times.

RB Bent Row

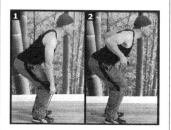

Step on the rubber band with one foot (easy difficulty) or both feet (hard difficulty). Grasping the rubber band in both hands, squat down slightly and bend your torso at 45° from the ground. Pull your elbows along your ribs toward your back, pause, then gradually return to the start position. You may have to grasp lower on the rubber band when you need more resistance.

RB Curl

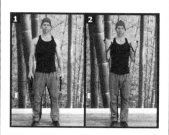

Step on the rubber band with one foot (easy difficulty) or both feet (hard difficulty). Grasping the rubber band in both hands at hip level, secure your elbows into your ribs and keep your posture erect. Bend at the elbows and bring your palms up to your shoulders, pause, then gradually return to start position.

RB Curl with Static Squat

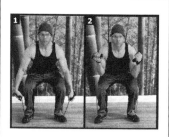

Step on the rubber band with both feet. Grasping the rubber band in both hands at hip level, secure your elbows into your ribs and come to a squatted position. Bend at the elbows and bring your palms up to your shoulders, pause, then gradually return to start position. Continue squatting for the entire exercise set.

RB Front Pulldown

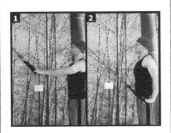

Attach the rubber band to a safe and secure position above your head. Stagger your stance, step back and straighten your arms out as you create full tension in the band. Start with your arms straight in front of your shoulders, then drive your arms down toward your hips. Aim your thumbs to your pockets. Pause, then slowly release back to the start position.

RB Hammer Curl

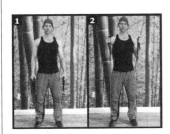

Step on the rubber band with one foot (easy difficulty) or both feet (hard difficulty). Grasping the rubber band in both hands at hip level, secure your elbows into your ribs and keep your posture erect. Bend at the elbows and bring your thumbs up to your shoulders, pause, then gradually return to start position.

RB High Pulldown

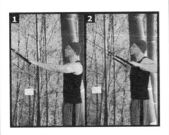

Attach the rubber band to a safe, secure position above your head. Stagger your stance, step back and straighten your arms out as you create full tension in the band. Slowly pull back your elbows at shoulder level, keeping your palms faced down. Pause, then gradually release your hold.

RB High Pulldown with Static Squat

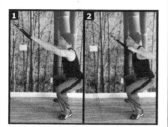

Attach the rubber band to a safe, secure position above your head. Step back, straighten your arms with full tension in the band and come to a squatted position. With your knuckles upward, pull your elbows in line with your shoulders (away from your ribs) to back behind you. Pause, then release your hold. Continue squatting for the entire exercise set.

RB Pulldown

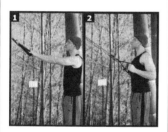

Attach the rubber band to a safe, secure position overhead. Stagger your stance, step back and straighten your arms out as you create full tension in the rubber band. Squeeze your elbows back behind you, pause, then gradually release your hold.

RB Reverse Fly

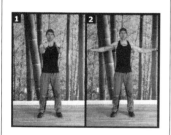

Grasp one end of the rubber band in each hand, extend your arms in front of your shoulder and wrap the excess tubing around your palms. With your palms facing down, extend your arms from the front to the outside of your shoulders. Pause, then return your arms back to the start position.

RB Rotation

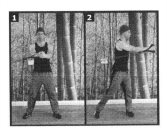

Firmly attach a rubber band at sternum level and turn your body with one side facing the wall. Stand a couple of feet away from the wall with shoulder-width stance. With both hands grasping the rubber band, extend your arms together in front of the sternum. Rotate your trunk away from the wall, pop up the inside heel and pivot on the toes. Pause in the furthest position, then return to the start. After the set is complete, switch directions to train both sides equally.

RB Row

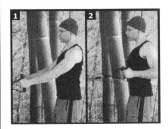

Attach the rubber band to a safe, secure position at hip level. Stagger your stance, step back and straighten your arms out as you create full tension in the band. Slide your elbows along your ribs to back behind you. Pause, then release your hold.

RB Row with Static Squat

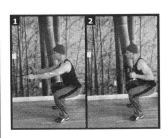

Attach the rubber band to a safe, secure position at hip level. Step back, straighten your arms with full tension in the band and come to a squatted position. Slide your elbows along your ribs to back behind you. Pause, then release your hold. Continue squatting for the entire exercise set.

RB Side Lunge with Rotation

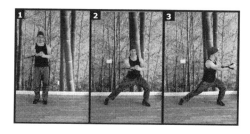

Firmly attach a rubber band at sternum level and turn your body with one side facing the attachment point. Stand a couple of feet away from the wall with a close-foot stance. With both hands grasping the rubber band, extend your arms together in front of the sternum. The foot closest to the attachment point stays planted as the other steps to the side. As you plant your foot down, squat that leg to 90° at the hip and knee, then rotate your trunk away from the attachment point. Pop up the inside heel and pivot on the toes. Pause in the furthest position, then return to the start. Repeat the movement sequence on the other side.

RB Side Raise

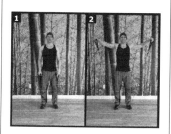

Step on the rubber band with one foot (easy difficulty) or both feet (hard difficulty). Grasping the rubber band in both hands at hip level, raise your straightened arms with knuckles up to shoulder level. Pause, then lower the weights back to your sides.

Helpful Tip: Inspect your rubber band before every workout to ensure there are no tears or rips. Safety first!

RB Triceps Extension

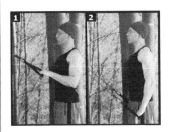

Attach the rubber band to a safe, secure position overhead. Stagger your stance, step back and straighten your arms out as you create full tension in the band. Tuck your elbows into your ribs, then drive your palms toward your hips. Bring your thumbs to your pockets. Pause, then slowly release the hold back to start position.

Reverse Crunch with Leg Extension

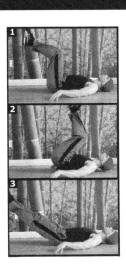

Lie on your back, place your arms out to your sides with your palms on the floor. Draw your legs to 90° bend at the hips, knees and ankles. Begin by lifting your butt off the ground and bringing your knees toward your head. Pause at the highest position you can, lower your legs to the start position, then extend your legs 45° from the ground. Return to the start position, then repeat the movement sequence.

Helpful Tip: Avoid placing your hands under your butt. This is a cheat method that will not help you build a good body. Work hard for your results. If your low back lifts off the floor, aim your feet higher. When you need more of a challenge, aim your feet lower to the ground. No butt tucking allowed!

Reverse Crunch with Rotation

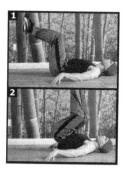

Lie on your back, place your arms out to your sides with your palms on the floor. Draw your legs to 90° bend at the hips, knees and ankles. Begin by lifting one side of your butt off the ground and bringing your knees toward your head. Pause at the highest position you can, then lower your legs to the start position. Repeat this movement sequence on the other side.

Reverse Crunch

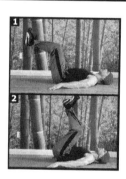

Lie on your back, place your arms out to your sides with your palms on the floor. Draw your legs to 90° bend at the hips, knees and ankles. Begin by lifting your butt off the ground and bringing your knees toward your head. Pause at the highest position you can, then lower your legs to the start position.

Helpful Tip: When "Reverse Crunches" are too difficult, stick with a more basic exercise like "Lying Leg Extensions." They target the same area and are as effective as "Reverse Crunches."

Reverse Hug

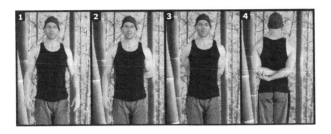

Reach both arms behind you and grasp your forearms as close to your elbows as possible. Pinch your shoulders back and down.

Reverse Lunge with Knee Up

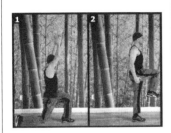

Separate your feet shoulder-width apart and place your hands on your hips. Step back with one leg, bend at both knees. Pop up the rear heel and bring the knee close to the ground. Focus on a 90° bend in the front knee. Press your rear foot off the ground while driving your front heel down to bring yourself back to a standing position. As you come to a standing position, bring the rear knee up in front of your hip.

Helpful Tip: If you are unable to do "Reverse Hug," try loosening up with the "Shoulder (wall)" stretch before you do it. This exercise will limber you up and make the "Reverse Hug" much easier.

Reverse Lunge with Knee Up

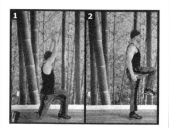

Separate your feet shoulder-width apart and place your hands on your hips. Step back with one leg, bend at both knees. Pop up the rear heel and bring the knee close to the ground. Focus on a 90° bend in the front knee. Press your rear foot off the ground while driving your front heel down to bring yourself back to a standing position. As you come to a standing position, bring the rear knee up in front of your hip.

Russian Twist with Bicycles

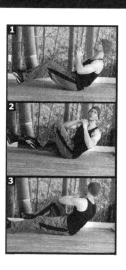

Come to a seated position on the ground with your knees bent and heels slightly lifted off the ground. Lean back onto your tailbone and clasp your hands in front of your sternum with your elbows bent. Rotate your torso to the left and bring your right knee up to meet your right elbow. Repeat this movement sequence in the opposite direction.

Helpful Tip: The "Russian Twist" is hard enough on its own, so adding bicycles to it makes it difficult. Experts only!

Russian Twist

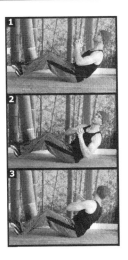

Come to a seated position on the ground with your knees bent and heels planted. Lean back onto your tailbone and clasp your hands in front of your sternum with your elbows bent. Rotate your torso to the left then to the right. Slowly repeat this movement sequence for the set.

Scissors

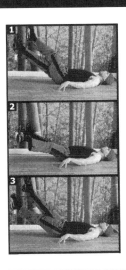

Lie on your back with your arms extended out to the side and palms placed on the ground. Draw your legs together and up 45° from the floor (or higher for decreased difficulty). Separate your legs as far apart as possible, then cross them over each other. Repeat this movement sequence while keeping your low back flat against the floor.

Seated Hamstring

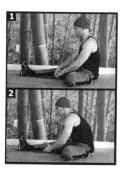

From a seated position, extend one leg out and tuck the other foot into your knee. Keep your posture erect as your reach to the extended leg and hold position. Change direction and stretch the opposite side for equal time.

Seated Knee Hug

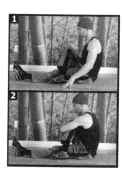

From a seated position, tuck one foot under the other leg with your heel next to the opposite buttock. Bring the top leg over the bent leg and place your heel next to the opposite leg. Hug your knee and hold position momentarily. Then, turn your torso toward the direction of the knee, place your arm into the ground look over your shoulder. Change direction and stretch the opposite side for equal time.

Helpful Tips for Better Stretching:
1. *Stretch until it's slightly uncomfortable, not painful*
2. *Breathe slowly and deeply*
3. *Focus on the area being stretched; try to relax it*
4. *Challenge yourself each stretch by going a little deeper*

Self Hug

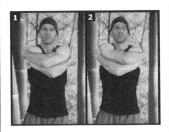

Cross your arms over your chest and hug yourself. Switch arm placement for an equal stretch.

Shoulder (wall)

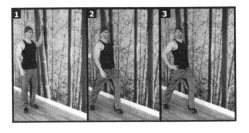

Stand within arm's reach of a wall to your side. Keep your posture upright at all times. On the side closest to the wall place your elbow (hand pointed upward) into the wall just outside of the side of your shoulder. With the foot closest the wall, step forward while keeping the heel of the back leg firmly planted. Pinch your shoulder blades back and turn your torso slightly away from the wall. Turn your head away from the wall. Change direction and stretch the opposite side for equal time.

Helpful Tip: Stretching is great any day of the week, even if it's your rest day.

Shoulder Roll

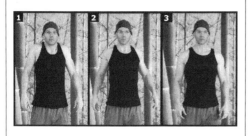

Bring your shoulders up, rotate them back, down then forward. Repeat this sequence for the entire exercise set. Change direction and stretch the opposite side for equal time.

Shoulder with Straight Arm (wall)

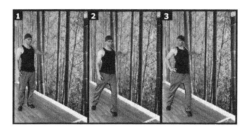

Stand within arm's reach of a wall to your side. Keep your posture upright at all times. On the side closest to the wall place your palm into the wall just outside of the side of your shoulder. With the foot closest the wall, step forward while keeping the heel of the back leg firmly planted. Pinch your shoulder blades back and turn your torso slightly away from the wall. Turn your head away from the wall. Change direction and stretch the opposite side for equal time.

Helpful Tip: Feeling tension in your upper back and neck? Try stretching your shoulders and chest area. Sometimes this tightness occurs from how you carry yourself throughout the day—especially if you work an office job.

Shuttle Run

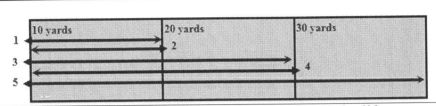

Shuttle runs require a 30-yard space that is marked off by a start position and 3 separate 10 yard increments. Sprint (run fast) from start position to the 10-yard position and back, then race from the start position to the 20-yard position and back. Lastly, burst from the start position to the 30-yard position and back. Touch each marked position or marker to indicate completion of each station sprint.

Side Bend

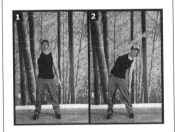

From a standing position, extend one arm directly overhead with your bicep by your ear. Keep your other arm directly at your side and bend your body directly to that side. Allow the downward arm to slide along the side of your thigh until your reach your full range of motion. Squeeze your mid-section and bring your body upright.

Words of Caution: If you become breathless while doing "Shuttle Runs," then slow down your pace. You never want to push yourself so hard that you cause bodily harm.

Side Crunch

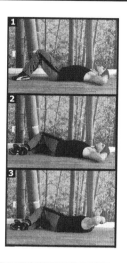

Lie on your back with your knees bent together and feet placed on the floor. Rotate your torso and bring both knees together to rest on the floor while keeping your shoulders flat on the ground. Place your fingertips behind your head and pull your elbows back. Press your ribs upward, pause, then lower yourself. Repeat the movement sequence for the entire exercise set and train each side equally.

Side Lunge

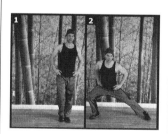

Start with your feet together and your arms loosely hanging at your sides. Step one foot to the side while keeping the other leg straight, squat down on the lead leg at a 90° bend in the hip and knee. Press off on the heel of your lead leg and come back to the start position.

Helpful Tip: Be sure that you get your butt down low as you can in the "Side Lunge." However, don't go down so far that you cause knee or hip issues. Imagine stepping to the side as if sitting on a chair.

Side Lying Leg Lift

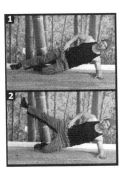
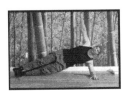

Lie on one side with your bottom knee bent and your top leg straightened. Place your bottom elbow into the ground with your forearm and palm placed flat to support and balance. Begin by lifting your top leg toward the ceiling while keeping your foot parallel to the ground. Lower that leg to the ground without touching, then repeat the movement sequence. Train each side equally.

Side Planks

With your leg together, lie on one side with your left elbow bent 90° and forearm placed away from you onto the floor. Pop your hip up to the ceiling and point your free arm toward the ceiling. Keep your body straight from your ankles to your shoulders. After holding this position for a set, switch to the other side and train equally.

Helpful Tip: For a challenge in "Side Planks," support yourself on a straightened arm. Once you master that modification, lift your top leg and hold.

For a less difficult modification, bend your bottom leg and support yourself on your knee. Bring your top arm down and assist with balance.

Side to Side Crunch

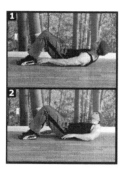

Lie on your back and place your feet flat on the ground with your knees bent. Press your ribs upward, pause at your highest position, then slowly reach with one arm to the same side heel and come back. Repeat the movement sequence as you reach to the other side.

Single Calf (pike)

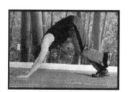

From a standing position, bend at the waist and place your palms into the ground. Keep your posture neutral and your butt faced to the ceiling. Your body should form a perfect triangle with the ground. Lift one leg and cross the foot over the back of your weight-bearing ankle. Hold. Stretch the opposite side for equal time.

Fun Facts: You never know your strength until you try an exercise. Additionally, you won't know your flexibility until you try a stretch.

Most times, people are unaware of how tight they are until they do a stretch. That is when they realize they are not as well off as they originally thought.

Single Leg Dynamic Bridge

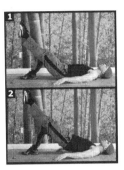

Lie on the ground with your arms out to the sides, knees bent and your feet placed flat on the floor. Extend one leg 45° from the ground. Begin by pressing your pelvis up and hold when your torso is 45° from the floor. Pause, squeeze your butt and tighten your abs for a 3-count, then gradually lower your butt back to the ground. Repeat this movement sequence and train each side equally.

Single Shoulder/Elbow Grasp

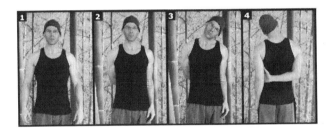

With one arm at your side, reach the other arm behind your back, and grasp the opposite elbow. Tilt your head away from the rear-positioned arm. Change direction and stretch the opposite side for equal time.

Fun Fact: Amazon warehouses have their employees stretch twice per shift—once at the beginning of the shift and another time after lunch break. And, there is no skipping this mandatory exercise requirement.

Skater Hop

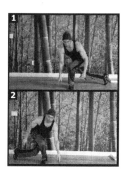

Establish a center line for you to use for this exercise and assume a slightly squatted stance. Hop to your left foot and draw your right foot over the line without touching the ground. Immediately, jump to your right and bring your left foot over the line without touching. Rapidly repeat this movement sequence.

Soccer Tap

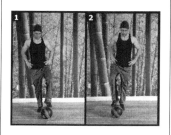

Equipment is not necessary though a ball can be helpful for those lacking imagination. From a standing position hop from one foot to the next, allowing your raised foot to gently toe-kick a "ball". Rapidly repeat this movement sequence.

Helpful Tip: When you are excessively sore from a previous workout, take it easier than normal so your body has time to recover. It's okay to exercise back-to-back days, but remember to vary your intensity.

Prioritize what part of your body is most important for you to develop. Then, choose to exercise more intense on those days.

Squat Thrust

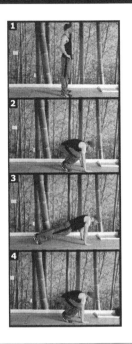

Start from a standing position with your hands on your hips, posture upright with your shoulder blades pinched back, chin up and your feet separated shoulder-width apart. Squat down and place your palms on the floor. Support your upper body weight on your palms as you pop your feet off the floor and extend your legs directly behind you. At this point explode your feet up again, drive your knees toward your chest and come back to the squatted position with your palms still flat on the floor. Squat up, place your hands on your hips, pinch your shoulder blades back and keep your chin up. Repeat this movement sequence and train each side equally.

Static Squat with Heel Raise

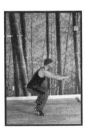

Squat down to a 90° bend in the hips and knees, then lift your heels off the ground. Hold this position for a timed set. The word "static" indicates a held position.

Don't limit your challenges, challenge your limits!

Static Squat

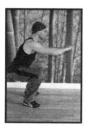

Squat down to a 90° bend in the hips and knees. The word "static" indicates a held position.

Stationary Jog

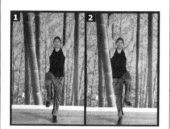

Bring your arms parallel above your head and jog in place. Drive your knees high.

Superman

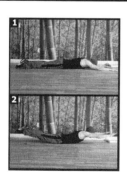

Lie flat on your stomach with your arms extended above your head. Lift your straightened arms and legs upward, pause then gradually lower them to the ground.

Trunk Rotation

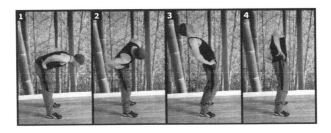

From a standing position, place your hands on your hips. Bend at the waist as far forward as you can go. Then slowly rotate from one side to the other.

Wall Chair with Toe Tap

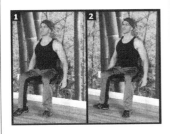

Come down to a squatted position with your back flat against a wall. Hold this position and tap your toes up and down. Avoid bracing, so keep your arms crossed or at your sides.

Wall Chair

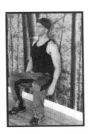

Come down to a squatted position with your back flat against a wall. Hold this position for a set time.

Wall Climber

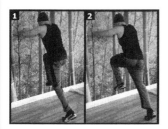

Step out from a wall about 3-4 feet, lean forward and place your hands on the wall. Begin by rapidly driving your legs up and in a jogging fashion, getting your knees high.

Window Wiper with Legs Extended

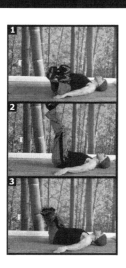

Lie on your back and place your extended arms to your sides for support. Begin with your legs straightened, pointing upward. Slowly rotate at the torso toward one direction, bringing your knees together toward the ground. Squeeze your abdomen and draw your knees back to start position. Repeat the movement sequence in the other direction.

Helpful Tip: Master the "Window Wiper" before progressing to the more difficult version with legs extended. This movement should be done slow as possible. Concentrate on engaging your abs every time you pull your legs back up toward the ceiling.

Window Wiper

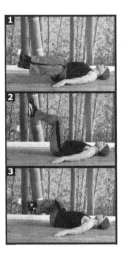

Lie on your back and place your extended arms to your sides for support. Begin with your legs bent 90° at the hips, knees and ankles. Slowly rotate at the torso toward one direction, bringing your knees together toward the ground. Squeeze your abdomen and draw your knees back to start position. Repeat the movement sequence in the other direction.

NOTE FROM THE AUTHOR

Reading an exercise is much easier than doing it. You may stumble over some instruction or need further clarification. I encourage you to contact me should you have any questions or comments.

It means a lot to me that you invested your time and money into my literature. So, I want you to get the most value as possible. The last thing I want to happen is for you to leave with questions.

The best part about sending me your questions, I can cover these questions in future publications. And, I would even be willing to put you into my special thanks section (permitting your approval).

Send your questions to me directly at ptdale@gmail.com. I answer all of my emails and am ecstatic when I hear from you. No matter the question or concern, drop me a line.

-Dale L. Roberts

Conclusion

The 90-day home workout plan is designed to maximize the most out of your exercise time while using a space with where you are familiar. The 5 components of a workout give the most comprehensive approach to your fitness. Each component has a vital part in your fitness growth, so take time to study your specific day's routine and the instructions for each exercise.

Component 1 is a great warm-up to get the body prepared for your routine so that you can perform all the exercises safely and prevent injury. Pick up the pace as you go into cardio training. Component 2 is to develop your cardio-respiratory endurance which helps train your heart. Weight training, component 3, develops and builds your body's muscle so that you not only look good, but feel good. Core training, component 4, is for strengthening the mid-section and support of your entire body. Slow down during this portion of the routine, so that you can begin your recovery. The last component, stretching, is to begin to loosen your muscles and to fully recover from your routine.

The first couple of weeks into the program, you may be a little sore, but if you stay consistent with your efforts this will subside. Feel free to use any of the stretches outside of your workouts to alleviate any extra tight areas. Keep yourself well-hydrated and eat good, whole foods to recover faster.

When you finish the first 90 days, you can rinse and repeat, but this time, measure your progress from your first 90 days. Tally your completed repetitions for your exercises on your first session, then compare it to the beginning of your second round of the 90-day plan. It's always exciting to see a marked improvement. It'll be further encouraging to take pictures at the beginning, then every 30 days after that. You'll get some excellent visual proof of your progress.

In the meantime, pick your start day, study your first week of workouts, then hit the ground running into the 90-day Home Workout Plan, your total body fitness program!

My Gratitude & Contact Info

Thank you for downloading my book. I hope you enjoyed it and found many insightful things. If it wouldn't be a bother, could you post an honest review of this book at Amazon.com? I read all of my reviews and really appreciate the open feedback so that I can continue to provide better books for you.

I'm not all about selling you my books—I do want to see you use what you've learned to build greater health and wellness. As you work toward your goals, however, you may have questions or run into some issues. I'd like to be able to help you, so let's connect. I don't charge for the assistance, so feel free to connect through any of the facets below:

On the web:

DaleLRoberts.com

Like me on Facebook:

http://www.facebook.com/authordaleroberts

Follow me on Twitter:

http://www.twitter.com/ptdaleroberts

Subscribe to my YouTube channel:

http://www.youtube.com/ptdalelroberts

Thank you, again! I hope to hear from you and wish you the best.

-Dale

About The Author

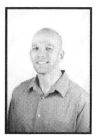

My name is Dale Lewis Roberts and I'm an American Council on Exercise Personal Trainer, Certified, with an ACE Specialty Certification in Senior Fitness. Since beginning my personal training career in 2006, I have earned numerous certifications in personal training, yoga, nutritional coaching, among others. I have worked with hundreds of clients with a variety of health & fitness goals.

While my greatest passions are health & fitness, writing and reading, I also love to spend time traveling with my wife, watching pro wrestling and playing guitar. I currently reside in Phoenix, Arizona, with my wife, Kelli, and our rescue cat, Izzie.

Subscribe to my blog at DaleLRoberts.com for all the latest posts on health and fitness tips. This is also one of the best ways to connect with me directly. Please, remember that whatever you do in life, make sure that you do what you love. Stay happy, healthy and strong!

Check out my collection of books at DaleLRoberts.com/my-book-shelf/.

ATTENTION: Get Your Free Gift

Are you interested in learning about the ten best fitness tools in fat loss? You are not alone! Millions of people all over the world are trying to lose weight and do so in a safe and effective manner.

What I have done is put together a FREE report to get you started on the road to success. This report won't be up forever, so get them before they are taken down. It's my simple way of saying thank you for buying this book.

http://DaleLRoberts.com/tenbest

Download the report on "The Ten Best Fitness Tools (To Get You More Results in the Least Time)" ABSOLUTELY FREE. The tips in this report will help you lose weight, melt off fat, and get in great shape!

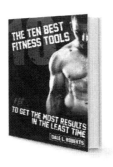

References

[1] The American Council on Exercise. (2015). Fit Facts/Exercise Programs/Warm Up to Work Out. Retrieved from http://www.acefitness.org/acefit/fitness-fact-article/2629/warm-up-to-work-out/

[2] The American Council on Exercise. (2015). Fit Facts: Monitoring Exercise Intensity Using Ratings of Perceived Exertion. Retrieved from http://www.acefitness.org/fitfacts/pdfs/fitfacts/itemid_2579.pdf

[3] Mayo Clinic Staff. (2014, February 5). Functional fitness training: Is it right for you? Retrieved from http://www.mayoclinic.org/healthy-living/fitness/in-depth/functional-fitness/art-20047680

[4] McCall, Pete. (2013, October 28). Recovery: The Forgotten Training Variable. Retrieved from http://www.acefitness.org/acefit/healthy-living-article/59/3581/recovery-the-forgotten-training-variable/

[5] Dalleck, Lance C. (2012, August). Training Recovery: The Most Important Component of Your Client's Exercise Program. Retrieved from http://www.acefitness.org/certifiednewsarticle/2757/training-recovery-the-most-important-component-of/

[6] Delaney, Bindi. (2013, October 11). Muscles of the Core. Retrieved from http://www.acefitness.org/blog/3562/muscles-of-the-core

[7] Freedman, Lisa. (2015). 5 Ways to Cool Down After a Workout. Retrieved from http://www.mensfitness.com/training/build-muscle/5-ways-to-cool-down-after-a-workout

[8] The American Council on Exercise. (2015). ACE's Top Ten Reasons to Stretch. Retrieved from http://www.acefitness.org/updateable/update_display.aspx?pageID=520

[9] The American Council on Exercise. (2015). ACE's Top Ten Reasons to Stretch. Retrieved from http://www.acefitness.org/updateable/update_display.aspx?pageID=520

[10] Stern, Denise. (2013, October 21). Shortness of Breath When Working Out. Retrieved from http://www.livestrong.com/article/306575-shortness-of-breath-when-working-out/

[11] Roshini, Raj. (2014, December 29). Dizzy During Workouts? When to See a Doctor. Retrieved from http://news.health.com/2014/12/29/dizzy-during-workouts-when-to-see-a-doctor/

[12] Madell, Robin. (2012, April 10). Signs of Heart Problems During Exercise. Retrieved from http://www.healthline.com/health/heart-disease/problems-during-exercise#1

[13] American Heart Association, Inc. (2015, March 25). Warning Signs of Heart Attack, Stroke or Cardiac Arrest. Retrieved from http://www.heart.org/HEARTORG/Conditions/911-Warnings-Signs-of-a-Heart-Attack_UCM_305346_SubHomePage.jsp

55765927R00080

Made in the USA
San Bernardino, CA
05 November 2017